T0201948

Psycho-Oncology in Palliative and End of Life Care

PSYCHO-ONCOLOGY CARE SERIES: COMPANION GUIDES
FOR CLINICIANS
Edited by Maggie Watson, PhD, and David W. Kissane, MD

Published and Forthcoming Books in the Psycho-Oncology Care Series
Management of Clinical Depression and Anxiety
Sexual Health, Fertility, and Relationships in Cancer Care
Psycho-Oncology in Palliative and End of Life Care
Cancer Survivorship and Health Promotion

Psycho-Oncology in Palliative and End of Life Care

Edited by

David W. Kissane, MD

Chair of Palliative Medicine Research, School of Medicine,
University of Notre Dame Australia and Cunningham Centre for
Palliative Medicine Research, St Vincent's Hospital Sydney, NSW;
Emeritus Professor of Psychiatry, Cabrini Health and Monash
Health, Monash University, Melbourne, VIC, Australia

Maggie Watson, PhD

Honorary Professor, Research Department of Clinical, Health
and Educational Psychology, University College London, UK;
Honorary Research Associate, Genetics and Epidemiology,
Institute of Cancer Research, Sutton and London, UK; Adjunct
Professor of Psychology, Research and Innovation, University of
Southern Queensland, Australia

William S. Breitbart, MD

Chairman, Jimmie C Holland Chair in Psychiatric Oncology,
Department of Psychiatry & Behavioral Sciences, Memorial Sloan
Kettering Cancer Center, New York, NY, USA;
Professor of Clinical Psychiatry, Weill Medical College of Cornell
University, New York, NY, USA

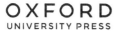
OXFORD
UNIVERSITY PRESS

OXFORD
UNIVERSITY PRESS

Oxford University Press is a department of the University of Oxford. It furthers
the University's objective of excellence in research, scholarship, and education
by publishing worldwide. Oxford is a registered trade mark of Oxford University
Press in the UK and certain other countries.

Published in the United States of America by Oxford University Press
198 Madison Avenue, New York, NY 10016, United States of America.

Library of Congress Cataloging-in-Publication Data
Names: Kissane, David W. (David William), editor. | Watson, M., editor. |
Breitbart, William, 1951- editor.
Title: Psycho-oncology in palliative and end of life care /
[edited by] David W. Kissane, Maggie Watson, William S. Breitbart.
Other titles: Psycho-oncology care.
Description: New York, NY : Oxford University Press, [2023] |
Series: Psycho oncology care |
Includes bibliographical references and index. |
Identifiers: LCCN 2022035038 (print) | LCCN 2022035039 (ebook) |
ISBN 9780197615935 (paperback) | ISBN 9780197615959 (epub) |
ISBN 9780197615966
Subjects: MESH: Neoplasms–psychology | Palliative Care | Terminal Care |
Professional-Patient Relations
Classification: LCC RC271.P33 (print) | LCC RC271.P33 (ebook) | NLM QZ 260 |
DDC 616.99/4029–dc23/eng/20220826
LC record available at https://lccn.loc.gov/2022035038
LC ebook record available at https://lccn.loc.gov/2022035039

DOI: 10.1093/med/9780197615935.001.0001

This material is not intended to be, and should not be considered, a substitute for
medical or other professional advice. Treatment for the conditions described in this
material is highly dependent on the individual circumstances. And, while this material
is designed to offer accurate information with respect to the subject matter covered
and to be current as of the time it was written, research and knowledge about medical
and health issues is constantly evolving and dose schedules for medications are being
revised continually, with new side effects recognized and accounted for regularly.
Readers must therefore always check the product information and clinical procedures
with the most up-to-date published product information and data sheets provided by
the manufacturers and the most recent codes of conduct and safety regulation. The
publisher and the authors make no representations or warranties to readers, express
or implied, as to the accuracy or completeness of this material. Without limiting the
foregoing, the publisher and the authors make no representations or warranties as to
the accuracy or efficacy of the drug dosages mentioned in the material. The authors
and the publisher do not accept, and expressly disclaim, any responsibility for any
liability, loss, or risk that may be claimed or incurred as a consequence of the use
and/or application of any of the contents of this material.

All case studies have been anonymized to protect patient identity.

9 8 7 6 5 4 3 2 1

Printed by Marquis, Canada

Preface

Psycho-oncology is a subspeciality of oncology that focuses on psychosocial problems experienced by cancer patients and their families; it provides evidence-based approaches to management of these specific problems.

These *Companion Guides in Psycho-Oncology Care* are intended to make clinical management information accessible to oncology clinical staff, psycho-oncologists, and allied professionals seeking to increase their psycho-oncology skills.

Mental health problems in cancer patients can be both preexisting and arise within the context of the cancer's diagnosis and treatment. This companion guide covers palliative and end of life care. As such, it brings the challenges of advanced cancer into sharp focus as the existential threat rises, bodily frailty can start to develop, and the person begins to face their mortality. The material presented here is intended for quick access by clinicians, whatever their discipline, as their patients and families face these challenges, whether medical, psychological, social, or spiritual in nature. Talking about dying is a poignant and sensitive task for every clinician and ought never to become easy, lest the person in need be not understood and accompanied with exquisite care. This care is directed not only to patients, but also their families, children and adolescents, culturally and linguistically diverse peoples, the bereaved, and the staff who care for all of these people—all of this is the remit of this book.

The authors of this *Companion Guide* are experienced clinicians and researchers with many years of experience in the care of patients with cancer and their families. We thank them for sharing this expertise. As editors, we also thank the staff of Oxford University Press for their support and the International Psycho-Oncology Society for their assistance with distribution of these official society clinical guides.

The psychosocial care of cancer patients and their families is a basic human right. We hope that the readers of this book will find it helpful to advance the quality of this care delivery to thus enrich the lives of all patients with cancer and their families.

David W. Kissane, MD
Maggie Watson, PhD
William S. Breitbart, MD

Contents

Contributors

Tatsuo Akechi, MD, PhD
Department of Psychiatry and
Cognitive-Behavioral Medicine,
Graduate School of Medical
Sciences, Nagoya City University,
Nagoya, Japan

Yesne Alici, MD, FACLP, FAPA
Psychiatry Service, Department
of Psychiatry and Behavioral
Sciences, Memorial Sloan
Kettering Cancer Center and
Weill Cornell Medical College,
New York, NY, USA

Allison J. Applebaum, PhD
Caregivers Clinic, Department
of Psychiatry and Behavioral
Sciences, Memorial Sloan
Kettering Cancer Center,
New York, NY, USA

Albert Balaguer, MD, PhD
School of Medicine and Health
Sciences, Universitat Internacional
de Catalunya, and Department
of Pediatrics at the Hospital
Universitari General de Catalunya.
Barcelona, Spain

Soenke Boettger, MD
Department of Psychosomatics and
Consultation-Liaison Psychiatry,
University Hospital Zurich,
University of Zurich, Zurich,
Switzerland

**William S. Breitbart, MD,
FACLP, DFAPA, FAPOS**
Department of Psychiatry & Behavioral
Sciences, Memorial Sloan Kettering
Cancer Center and Weill Medical
College of Cornell University,
New York, NY, USA

**Jayita Deodhar, MD, MRCPsych,
PGDipPallMed**
Tata Memorial Hospital and Homi
Bhabha National Institute,
Mumbai, Maharashtra, India

Maria Die Trill, PhD
Clínica Universidad de Navarra,
Madrid Site; Psycho-Oncology
Service, Department of
Medical Oncology, Madrid,
Spain; University of Salamanca,
Spain

Chun-Kai Fang, MD
Department of Psychiatry &
Hospice and Palliative Care
Center, MacKay Memorial
Hospital, Taipei, Taiwan

Daisuke Fujisawa, MD, PhD
Department of Neuropsychiatry
and Palliative Care Center,
Keio University School
of Medicine, Shinjuku-ku,
Tokyo, Japan

Luigi Grassi, MD, MPhil
Institute of Psychiatry, Department
of Neuroscience and
Rehabilitation, University of
Ferrara; St. Anna University
Hospital and Health Trust,
Ferrara, Italy

Melissa Henry, PhD
Faculty of Medicine, Gerald
Bronfman Department of
Oncology, McGill University;
Psycho-Oncology Research
Group, Lady-Davis Institute
for Medical Research, Jewish
General Hospital, Montreal,
QC, Canada

Brian Kelly, BMed, PhD, FRANZCP, FAChPM
Research and Innovation Division
   and School of Medicine and
   Public Health, University of
   Newcastle, Australia; Division of
   Psychosocial Oncology, Cumming
   School of Medicine, University of
   Calgary, Canada

David W. Kissane, AC, MD, BS, MPM, FRANZCP, FAChPM, FACLP
School of Medicine, University
   of Notre Dame Australia and
   Cunningham Centre for Palliative
   Medicine Research, St Vincent's
   Hospital Sydney, NSW; Cabrini
   Health and Monash Health,
   Monash University, VIC, Australia

Mark Lazenby, RN, PhD, FAAN, FAPOS
Sue & Bill Gross School of Nursing,
   University of California, Irvine,
   CA, USA

Wendy G Lichtenthal, PhD
Bereavement Clinic, Department of
   Psychiatry and Behavioral Sciences,
   Memorial Sloan Kettering Cancer
   Center, New York, NY, USA

Daniel McFarland, DO
Department of Medicine, Northwell
   Health Cancer Institute; Manhattan
   Eye Ear Throat Hospital/Lenox
   Hill Hospital, New York, NY;
   Department of Psychiatry,
   Memorial Sloan Kettering Cancer
   Center, New York, NY, USA

Natasha Michael, MB, ChB, MSc, FRACP, FAChPM
Palliative and Supportive Care
   Department, Cabrini Health;
   School of Medicine, Sydney
   Campus, University of Notre
   Dame Australia, Darlinghurst,
   NSW; Faculty of Medicine,
   Nursing and Health Sciences,
   Monash University, VIC, Australia

Hannah-Rose Mitchell, PhD, MPH
Department of Psychiatry and
   Behavioral Sciences, Memorial
   Sloan Kettering Cancer Center,
   New York, NY, USA

Christian Ntizimira, MD, MMSc
African Center for Research on
   End of Life Care, Rwanda; Kofi
   Annan Global Health Leadership
   Programme, Palliative Care
   Center for Excellence in Research
   and Education (PalC), Singapore

Cristina Monforte-Royo, RN, MSN, PhD
Department of Nursing, School of
   Medicine and Health Sciences,
   Universitat Internacional de
   Catalunya, Barcelona, Spain

Robert A. Neimeyer, PhD
Department of Psychology,
   University of Memphis, Portland
   Institute for Loss and Transition,
   Portland, OR, USA

Crystal Park, PhD
Department of Psychological
   Sciences, University of
   Connecticut, Storrs, CT, USA

William F. Pirl, MD, MPH
Department of Psychosocial
   Oncology and Palliative Care,
   Dana-Farber Cancer Institute,
   Boston, MA; Harvard Medical
   School, Boston, MA, USA

Josep Porta-Sales, MD, PhD
School of Medicine and Health
   Sciences, Universitat Internacional
   de Catalunya, and Palliative
   Care Service at Institut Català
   d'Oncologia, Barcelona, Spain

William E. Rosa, PhD
Department of Psychiatry and
   Behavioral Sciences, Memorial
   Sloan Kettering Cancer Center,
   New York, NY, USA

Rajvi Shah, MB, BS
Supportive, Psychosocial and Palliative
    Care Research Department,
    Cabrini Health, VIC, Australia;
    School of Medicine, University
    of Notre Dame Australia,
    Darlinghurst, NSW, Australia

Jane Turner, MBBS, PhD, FRANZCP
Discipline of Psychiatry, The
    University of Queensland, K
    Floor, Mental Health Centre,
    Herston, QLD, Australia

Yosuke Uchitomi, MD, PhD
National Cancer Center Institute
    for Cancer Control, Chuo-ku,
    Tokyo, Japan

Maggie Watson, PhD, Dip.Clin. Psych.
Research Department of Clinical,
    Health and Educational
    Psychology, University
    College London; Genetics
    and Epidemiology, Institute
    of Cancer Research, Sutton,
    UK; Research and Innovation,
    University of Southern
    Queensland, Australia

Talia Zaider, PhD
Family Therapy Clinic, Department
    of Psychiatry and Behavioral
    Sciences, Memorial Sloan
    Kettering Cancer Center,
    New York, NY, USA

Chapter 1

Communication about Advanced Progressive Disease, Prognosis, and Advance Care Plans

Natasha Michael and Rajvi Shah

Learning Objectives

After reading this chapter, the clinician will be able to:

1. Appreciate the communication challenges patients, families, and health professionals face in advanced cancer, strategies to assist, and the importance of maintaining hope.
2. Recognize and implement approaches for communicating disease progression, recurrence, and transition to palliative care.
3. Understand the importance of prognostication in cancer, options for formulating prognosis and effective ways to communicate prognosis.
4. Recognize the importance of family communication and recommended styles of facilitating a family meeting.
5. Take account of significant cultural, ethical, and legal considerations for communication.
6. Know how to define and execute advance care planning in cancer.

Background Evidence

Communication in Cancer and Its Importance

A diagnosis of cancer devastates families, commonly precipitating an existential crisis and adjustment challenges. A fundamental disruption occurs to the psychosocial aspects of one's life, with a loss of predictability, disruption of ambition and plans, and the heralding of uncertainty. Families are affected as a unit of care rather than as isolated individuals, raising unique communication challenges. Consideration is required as to each individual and their family's strengths and vulnerabilities, coping, and capacity to adjust to information.

Communication is central to our human existence and forms the basis of every therapeutic encounter. For a patient with advanced cancer, the content, method, and communication circumstances are central to achieving the common goal of realizing the best possible length and quality of life. Poor communication from diagnosis to death commonly evokes anxiety and despair for those who seek clarity, openness, and honesty, with timely information delivered sensitively and relationally.[1]

Patients and families commonly describe the following experiences in cancer communication:

- Lack of warning of impending bad news in a consultation
- Use of terminology or language that is not readily understood
- Too much verbal information provided causing difficulty in retention
- Important information on diagnosis and prognosis relayed too late in the disease
- Clinicians' reluctance to discuss prognosis or be honest about the potential for treatment failure
- Lack of respect for cultural or personal variations in beliefs or communication styles

Health professionals face equal challenges in cancer communication, which commonly trigger personal distress and subsequent burnout. Common communication challenges faced by professionals include:

- Maintaining hope while imparting complex information
- Finding the appropriate language to divulge technical and medical information clearly
- Empowering patients to participate in shared decision-making
- Limited time and logistical challenges
- Coping with changes in therapeutics, technology, and investigative procedures

Effective communication (see Box 1.1) requires both knowledge and skills, with leading oncological institutions recommending skills-based communication training for all practitioners.[2]

Professional communication requires a readiness to communicate and openness. The "communication compass" model[3] (see Figure 1.1) describes the key elements, which consist of two axes:

- Associated perspectives of the clinician and the patient
- Content of information and emotional experience

The rapid changes occurring in cancer therapeutics pose challenges across both axes.[4] While the term "cancer" continues to evoke death anxiety from the patient's perspective, the continued offering of therapeutic interventions by the oncologist can create a "collusion of hope," thus causing a malalignment of perspectives between patients, families, and clinicians. Additionally, diagnostic and prognostic information provokes an emotional experience, which is individual, personal, and requires time, space, and recognition for adequate processing. Clarification of the emotional experience is essential to identify or

Box 1.1 Key Areas That Require Specific Expertise in Communication

- Breaking bad news—disclosing a diagnosis, disease recurrence, progression, and treatment failure
- Discussing prognosis and disease trajectory
- Communicating with family members and achieving concordance in communication
- Discussing clinical trials, novel cancer diagnostics, and therapeutics and ensuring informed consent
- Exploring and communicating about difficult emotional and psychoexistential issues
- Encouraging early integration of palliative care and benefits of psychological and social support
- Communicating with patients from diverse cultural and linguistic backgrounds, children, young adults, and the disenfranchised
- Negotiating withdrawal of treatment and preparation for end of life care
- Navigating interprofessional communication and conflict resolution within teams

prevent maladaptive responses, and ensure adequate psychological support is available to those who require it.

Communicating Information in Cancer

Communicating information to the patient starts with understanding their frame of reference. This includes exploring how they perceive their current

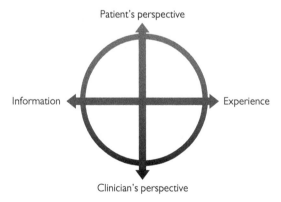

Figure 1.1 Communication compass.

Source: Reproduced with permission from Maex E, De Valck C. Key elements of communication in cancer care. In Stiefel F, Editor. Communication in Cancer Care. Berlin, Heidelberg: Springer-Verlag; 2006.

situation, and what they understand and know. Many patients fail to understand and recall information provided in consultations,[5] with studies suggesting that

- 40%–80% of medical information is forgotten immediately
- Over half the amount of information recalled may be incorrect
- The greater the amount of information the clinician presents, the lower the proportion correctly recalled by the patient

Studies have demonstrated the benefit of several strategies and tools to improve cancer communication and the retention of information. These include the use of question prompt lists, audio recordings of key consultations and provision of summaries for the patient, and for the clinician, communication skills training.

Question Prompt Lists

Question prompt lists (QPLs) are structured lists of fixed or optional questions provided by a service or a clinician to a patient prior to their consultation to help them prepare for it.[5] Please see an example of a QPL[6] commonly used in palliative care clinics in the Appendix of this book.

QPLs may benefit patients who struggle to formulate questions themselves by encouraging them to:

- Ask at least one question
- Increase the number of questions they might ask
- Ask difficult questions that may be forgotten or avoided

QPLs help to:

- Assist with addressing patient and caregiver information needs in the areas of diagnosis, investigations to complete, treatment options, and prognostication.
- Shifting the theme of a consultation toward a more appropriate area, e.g., disease trajectory, treatment options, and procedures in a hospital.

Studies have shown that QPLs do not increase consultation time, but the physician's active endorsement of a QPL may lead to better information recall. QPLs that lead to the exploration of personal or emotional issues may enable a stronger therapeutic alliance to be developed between patient and clinician.

Consultation Audio Recording and Written Summaries

Consultation audio recordings are digital recordings of medical consultations provided to the patient following a medical consultation.[7] Evidence supports the benefit of these recordings with patients reporting higher satisfaction levels and feeling enabled to participate in decision-making. Providing patients with a copy of the recording or a written summary allows for greater information recall, reduces anxiety, and enhances their perception of being adequately informed.

Patients should be provided with a choice as to whether to receive communication aids, recordings, or written summaries to ensure distress is minimized and personal preferences are met.

Communication Skills Training

Communication skills training is now mandatory for oncology and palliative care staff across several jurisdictions in a large number of countries. Practitioners personalities and individual beliefs, values, and cultural orientations can impact outcomes. Evidence has demonstrated the benefits of both group and online training in changing behaviors and attitudes.[8] Shorter duration training courses have been shown to be less successful than longer ones, with no apparent differences between actual or simulated patients.

An example of a communication skills training method would be the Comskil program,[9] which is located at Memorial Sloan-Kettering Cancer Center in New York. Delivery of news of recurrence and disease progression are basic for advanced cancer and well exemplified by the SPIKES approach,[10] a model that involves:

- **S**etting up—preparation, arrange for privacy and clarify the reason for consultation
- **P**erception—pick up on patient cues that may suggest anxiety about the future or vulnerability
- **I**nvitation—clarify the degree of details they want disclosed, invite questions
- **K**nowledge—provide information in small amounts, clarifying understanding
- **E**motions—recognize, normalize and empathize with patient emotions
- **S**trategy and **S**ummary—check understanding, summarize, and review next steps

Presenting Problems

Five types of presentation and their management will be considered in this chapter:

1. The patient with disease recurrence or progression;
2. The patient wanting to discuss prognosis;
3. The patient entering the terminal phase of life;
4. Communicating with family and caregivers;
5. When an advance care plan is needed.

Disease Recurrence or Progression

Communicating disease recurrence or progression requires preparation and thoughtfulness and, importantly, identifying the psychologically vulnerable patient (see Table 1.1) who may require specific considerations. The clinician should ensure that the patient is accompanied and supported when information about relapse or recurrence is provided.

The following case study describes how a vulnerable patient's denial of diagnosis and progression is used as a coping mechanism.

Table 1.1 Factors That May Indicate a Psychologically Vulnerable Patient or Family

Indicators of Patient Vulnerability	Indicators of Family Vulnerability
• Delay in presentation despite significant physical symptoms	• Family dysfunction through relationship breakdown, estrangement
• The use of denial as a coping mechanism	• Multiple traumatic losses within the family unit
• Significant history of mental health illnesses such as depression, anxiety, borderline personality disorder, and psychotic disorders	• Antagonistic and conflictual communication style
• History of somatization to cope with emotional distress	
• History of substance abuse, self-harming behavior	

Case Study 1

A 58-year-old female with lung cancer lives alone. A diagnosis of a hoarding disorder is apparent with the involvement of the community services. She is admitted to the hospital for pain, and functional decline and investigations confirm significant disease progression. She is reviewed by the junior physician, who requests that she consents to a Do Not Resuscitation order. The patient informs the doctor that she has a simple chest infection and wants to be discharged home. The physician repeatedly emphasizes the cancer diagnosis, progression, and poor prognosis. The patient becomes increasingly agitated, accusing the physician of trying to kill her, pulling out her intravenous cannula and attempting to run out of the hospital.

The above case illustrates how distress is induced by not being attuned to the patient's inability to accept her diagnosis and the underlying vulnerability. A more patient-centered approach allows the patient to feel more in control, with the physician first exploring what information the patient would like to receive.

How Much Time Do I Have? Communicating Prognosis

The prognosis is an estimate of the likely course and outcome of a disease. In cancer, it provides an estimation of success with treatment and chances of recovery. Prognostication is dynamic due to biological, clinical, and social factors beyond the diagnosis and stage of the disease.[11] An assessment of prognosis should thus be deliberate and explicit, and is central to communication success in advanced cancer.

Communication of prognostic information requires the communication of truthful information while maintaining hope. A proportion of patients may choose not to know their prognosis, with family members seeking more detailed information.

Why Is Prognostication Important?

For patients with advanced illnesses, accurate survival prediction is critical to enable personal, clinical, and ethical decision-making. Accurate prognostic information allows patients, their families and clinicians the opportunity to:

• Make plans and reorder life's priorities
• Consider decision-making around medical interventions, weighing risks and burdens against life expectancy and personal goals
• Set meaningful goals and expectations for care, including advance care planning, preferred place of care and death
• Address financial and legal affairs
• Explore support options available that rely on prognosis, e.g., access to hospice care, superannuation, and welfare benefits

Prognostication[11] involves two distinct skills, (1) the formulation, and then (2) the communication of this prognosis.

Formulation of Prognosis

The prognosis can be formulated either:

Subjectively: based on clinician intuition and prediction of survival
Objectively: using prognostic factors and models to determine an actuarial prediction of survival.

Subjective Formulation of Prognosis

Clinician prediction of survival (CPS) is the most common approach for estimating survival in cancer patients (see Table 1.2). CPS usually take one of three approaches:[11]

Table 1.2 Approaches Used in a Clinician's Prediction of Survival (adapted from Hui et al.[11])

Approach	Temporal Question	Surprise Question	Probabilistic Question
Question	How long will this patient live?	Would I be surprised if this patient died in (specific time frame)?	What is the probability of survival within a specific time frame?
Answer	Specific time frame	Yes or no	0% to 100% (at 10% increments)
Definition of an Accurate Response	If estimated time frame was +/ - 33% of actual survival	If "no" answer and patient died within a specific time frame; or If "yes" answer and patient remained alive by specified time frame	If answered ≤30% probability and patient died within specified time frame; or if answered ≥70% probability and patient remained alive by specified time frame
Accuracy	20%–30%	76%–88% (1 year time frame)	53%–91% (6 months to 24-hour time frames)

1. Temporal Prediction: How long will this patient live?
2. Probabilistic Prediction: What is the probability of survival of this patient in (specific time frame)?
3. Surprise Question Prompt: Would I be surprised if this patient dies in (specific time frame)?[11]

🔍 Key Point

Studies evaluating the accuracy of CPS in advanced cancer have found that clinician intuition can be inaccurate, with overall survival estimates incorrect by a factor of approximately 5.3 in the optimistic direction.[12]

Discussion and estimation within the multi-professional team can improve prognostic accuracy.

Objective Formulation of Prognosis

Clinical signs and symptoms and the use of laboratory variables may improve the accuracy of CPS. These may include:

The Karnofsky Performance Status and Palliative Performance Scale are widely used in the palliative care setting to assess and monitor changes to a patient's functional status. They require clinicians to match signs and symptoms of a patient's function to a description on a functional scale. These performance scales have been shown to correlate with survival in a variety of settings, with performance status known to decline in the months before death and a steeper deterioration occurring in the days and weeks prior to death.

Clinical predictors are sometimes combined through analytical weighting to produce a single patient score that is mapped to an expected survival, with extensive research confirming the benefit of using validated prognostic scores.[13] These include the

- Palliative Prognostic Index (PPI), which uses performance status and clinical signs and symptoms to create a regression model to predict survival.[13]

Box 1.2 Clinical Signs and Symptoms of Poor Prognosis in Advanced Cancer

Patient Factors
- Deterioration in performance status
- Delirium or cognitive failure
- Dyspnoea at rest
- Cancer anorexia-cachexia syndrome

Laboratory Variables
- Elevated CRP
- Hypoalbuminemia
- Leucocytosis
- Lymphopenia
- Hyponatremia
- Hypercalcemia

- Palliative Prognostic Score (PaP), which integrates a CPS score with five other criteria to predict 30-day survival.[13]
- Palliative Performance Scale (PPS), which estimates prognosis based on changes across five functional parameters.[13]

Communication of Prognosis

Following the formulation of prognosis, a clinician needs to decide what to communicate to those who seek information about their prognosis. However, clinicians can find this area challenging and commonly:

- Miss or avoid cues from patients who want to discuss prognosis
- Focus on treatment options and create false optimism
- Underestimate the patients' prognostic information needs
- Overestimate the patients' understanding of their illness and likely outcomes.

When to initiate and how to discuss prognostic information is highly individualized, with the information needs of patients differing and altering during the course of their illness. The content of prognostic information can vary and include life expectancy, expected treatment outcomes, adverse effects, bodily changes in the last weeks to days of life, and likely care needs.

Given prognostic uncertainty, for patients and families who would like a numerical estimation of their life expectancy, clinicians commonly use broad categories:

- "Days to weeks," or "hours to days," as opposed to a single point in time for life-expectancy, e.g., 48 hours or 2 months.
- Estimated survival can involve median survival curves of 6 months, and explaining typical, best- and worst-case scenarios.

Regardless of the scope and depth of prognostic information communicated, it is important for the clinician to acknowledge the patient and family's emotional response to the information and check their understanding of it. A summary of key steps in communicating prognosis is shown here in Box 1.3.

Box 1.3 Steps in Discussing Prognosis

- Prepare by determining prognostic parameters with and without life-prolonging treatment
- Alert patient that you will be discussing important aspects of their illness and recommend that they bring along a support person
- Clarify patient's understanding of their medical situation, information desired, and readiness to receive prognostic information
- Ensure all family members desire the same prognostic information (patients may sometimes choose not to know but caregivers may request information)
- Communication of information should ideally occur within a therapeutic relationship of trust
- Information should be consistent among members of the wider multidisciplinary team

Communicating about the Terminal Phase and End of Life Care

Talking about Dying

Communication at the end of life inevitably evokes an emotional response and warrants communication that addresses the biomedical and psychoexistential aspects of care to help patients transcend their suffering and despair. The primary concerns for many at this stage are the relationships with family and friends, seeking purpose, meaning, love, and forgiveness.[14] Thus, an essential aspect of talking about dying is focusing on "whole person care" to enable patients to transcend their suffering and despair.

Many clinicians are unexposed to formal training in this area and avoid direct conversations, use euphemisms, and avoid the exploration of the spiritual and psychoexistential.[14,15]

🔍 Key Point

Communication about the terminal phase can occur:

1. While the patient is still relatively well and forms part of an advance care planning discussion. Questions asked may provide insight into previous traumatic experiences of death and may include:
   • What will the end be like?
   • Will you be able to manage my pain, and how can I be sure I will not suffocate to death?
2. In the final weeks or days of life, when communication may be limited to short conversations and less dominated by the transmission of medical information. Communication at this stage focuses on
   • The nonverbal communication and attitude of the physician—moving from task-orientated behavior to care-orientated behavior
   • Importantly, clinicians have an essential role in simply being present in the moment and accompanying the dying patient

Additional information that may be communicated to patients and families are listed in Box 1.4.

🔍 Key Point: Strategies to Facilitate Hope during End of Life Discussions

It may seem paradoxical to discuss hope as one approaches the end of life, but hope is central to those facing an uncertain future and, therefore, of all communication within palliative care.[16] However, hope in this context can take various forms and range from hoping for a miraculous cure to a desire for a death free of pain and suffering. Clinicians can be a conduit for hope by acknowledging difficulties and communicating empathetically, using appropriate words and approaches. Useful strategies are found in Table 1.3.

Communicating with Caregivers and Families

The role of the family in the cancer patient's care has been augmented with the enhancement of care and death in the community setting. A cancer diagnosis affects the entire family and is a well-known contributor to family stress due to uncertainty about the future, loss of roles and routines,

Box 1.4 Issues to Communicate as a Patient Approaches the End of Life

- Confirm preferred place of death
  - Rapid discharge home from hospital can be facilitated, or some patients may prefer for death not to occur at home
- Explain the functional, physical, and care changes that may occur in the last few days of life
  - Eating and drinking less and sleeping more
  - Changes in breathing and pulse
  - Changes in color and temperature of the skin
  - Increased respiratory secretions
  - Acute confusion, or reduced conscious state, suggesting delirium
  - The possible need for the insertion of a catheter or use of a continuous infusion of medication
- Alleviate anxiety about the patient dying of starvation or thirst
  - Communicate and encourage the involvement of family in providing oral care to alleviate thirst
  - Listen attentively and consider use of low-volume subcutaneous fluids where families make a request for cultural or religious purposes
- Address any fears and myths about the process of dying
  - Explore any previous negative experiences of death
  - Address fears about dying in pain and the use of opioids
  - Reassure that support will be provided to family
- Being present with the dying
  - Establish the family's desire to be present for the last few days and hours of life
  - Reassure that no judgments are made about individual decisions
  - Provide practical advice around the availability of food and sleeping arrangements if family choose to remain by the bedside of the dying
  - Encourage the normalization of the dying process so that families feel relaxed in the environment
- Existential and spiritual needs
  - Address existential issues that the patient or family may articulate; fear of the dying process, feeling alone or abandoned, fear of the afterlife
  - Facilitate conflict resolution and reconciliation where possible within families
  - Offer pastoral support and establish the need for specific spiritual or religious support
- Care immediately after death
  - Provide information on what happens to the body after death, advice on funeral directors
  - Establish if there are specific religious or cultural practices that require observation
  - Clarify the process of death certification, autopsy if required, organ or tissue donation if requested

Table 1.3 Useful Strategies to Maintain Hope at the End of Life

Approach	Useful Strategies	Examples of Phrases to Use to Maintain Hope
Reassurance of physical and emotional comfort	Explain the benefits of best supportive care	"Though we cannot offer you anti-cancer treatment, patients who receive best supportive care and manage their pain and symptoms well can live longer with a better quality of life."
Advocate non-abandonment and ongoing caring relationships with the team	Emphasize the support structures available to the patient and family.	"You will be referred to the local community palliative care service who will visit you regularly and discuss your care at home with your doctors."
Encouraging self-worth and a sense of identity	Assist with reframing expectations to achieve meaningful outcomes	"Returning to work full-time may be a challenge. Have you considered negotiating working flexibly at reduced hours? This will allow a gradual return of your strength and confidence after you complete treatment."
Promote personal and family values	Encourage advance care planning and legacy work	"This time is for meaningful conversations with your family about the kind of care you want to receive, memory making, and seeing to your affairs. This can take a lot of pressure off your family."
Promote a sense of meaning and purposeful living until the end	Preserving who one is—a person's values, attitudes and life's intention—to the very end	"Receiving bad news does not mean we lose hope and a sense of who we are. I would encourage you to continue to draw from the things that have always helped you; your family and faith and your strong support network of friends."

financial strains, and existential concerns. Family caregivers suffer considerable anxiety and distress, which lead to poor coping and subsequent bereavement outcomes.[16] Family members can be described as inextricably linked individuals and may include direct blood relatives, friends and partners, or those with whom the patient feels most connected. As such, " 'family" can be whomever the patient nominates as "family."

Family-centered care is central to the philosophy of palliative care, is introduced in this chapter, and will be expanded in Chapter 7. In caring for the cancer patient, the family's involvement in information provision, decision-making, and future care planning improves both patient and caregiver outcomes. A seasoned practitioner aims to ensure triadic congruence in communication between the patient, caregiver, and clinician.

Family Meetings

Information to family members or significant others is best communicated through a family meeting, sometimes known as a family conference. Family meetings are an opportunity to identify a family's communication style and values. It is recommended that in advanced cancer, family meetings[17] should occur:

• During any period of transition, e.g., a change of treatment intent, withdrawal of disease-modifying treatment, or cessation of treatment

• To assist the family with the preparation for a declining trajectory, allow the opportunity for questions, and educate the family about the management of symptoms

• To identify members of the family who may need additional support. These may include those at risk of complex grief, and children or young adults who may need support.

• To discuss and prepare a family for discharge and care in the community

• Preparation for end of life care and care following death and into the bereavement period

A proactive approach should be undertaken to plan and execute these meetings (see Box 1.5), and meetings should not be reserved for "crisis situations."

Box 1.5 Steps to Undertake in Planning and Execution of a Family Meeting

• A nominated team member should identify participating family members and coordinate a time and place for a meeting.

• Offer the option of telehealth or online access for members of the family who are unable to attend in person.

• Explain to the patient and family the reason for the meeting and topics that will be discussed.

• Encourage them to prepare a list of questions they may want addressed or provide a template document that will enable them to list areas of concern prior to the meeting.

• Identify members of the multidisciplinary team or external members that may be required to attend. Consider invitation of a long-standing and involved general practitioner, mental health, or other professional for those with specific needs.

 Specific communication skills and techniques (see Table 1.4) can be used to obtain the best outcomes in a family meeting.[23]

Table 1.4 Specific Communication Skills and Techniques to Use in a Family Meeting (adapted from Coyle and Kissane[17])

Phase 1: *Clinician-led part* Goal: to educate, clarify, and plan for future care	Discuss medical illness, disease trajectory, current and future treatment options
Phase 2: *Psychosocial-led part* Goal: to explore the psychological and emotional impact of illness	Explore patient and family coping, different emotional responses, and the impact of illness on individuals and the family unit
Phase 3: Practicalities of discharge ongoing inpatient care.	Involve members of the multidisciplinary team. A pastoral practitioner may assist with discussing spiritual care before and after death and bereavement support
Question Styles to be Adopted in a Meeting	**Example of Questions**
Circular questions Preserves facilitator neutrality and encourages collaboration among family members in seeking solutions.	*"How do you think your father is coping since your mother was diagnosed with cancer?"*
Reflexive questions Encourages reflection on possibilities to improve family involvement and cohesion.	*"What may be the benefits of caring for your father at home rather than placing him in a nursing home?"*
Strategic questions Guides the family toward the best outcome for the patient.	*"What are the changes in your wife's condition that need to occur that may make you both think that it may be time to stop chemotherapy?"*
Summarizing family concerns The clinician maintains professional neutrality in reflecting the family's views, highlighting areas of concordance and discordance.	*"There is agreement that it is time to stop regular blood transfusions. You recognize the lack of benefit it provides but are understandably concerned that you may be 'giving up on your father.' These are commonly articulated concerns, but we draw comfort from your father's involvement in this decision and his desire to withdraw treatment at this point."*

Advance Care Planning in Advanced Cancer

🔍 Key Point

What Is It?

"Advance care planning is defined as a process that supports adults at any age or stage of health in understanding and sharing their personal values, life goals, and preferences regarding future medical care. The goal of advance care planning is to help ensure that people receive medical care that is consistent with their values, goals and preferences during serious and chronic illness."[18]

Advance care planning (ACP) is now identified as a key quality indicator in cancer care. It is best conceptualized as an opportunity to allow a cancer patient and their trusted persons to prepare for future healthcare and, if ready, meaningfully prepare for their dying. The process of ACP should ideally be

- Dynamic: a process that changes, evolves, and progresses over time
- Iterative: a process that requires multiple repeated conversations
- Longitudinal: occurring throughout the trajectory of illness
- Involve continuity: occur within an existing and continuing clinician relationship

Patients' wishes should be reviewed over time, especially during transition periods and with changing health states. Many cancer patients choose to have conversations but withhold formal documentation due to feeling unprepared, limited health literacy, or language barriers. Nonetheless, it is recommended any ACP conversation should be documented in the medical records to ensure alignment of care with the patient's values and preferences.

Case Study 2

Alan is a 42-year-old father of three young children and is married to Yvonne. Alan has been the primary provider for the family and runs his own gas fitting business.

He was diagnosed with early-stage pancreatic cancer 2 years ago and underwent a successful Whipple's procedure. He recovered well and completed adjuvant chemotherapy with no evidence of recurrent disease until 6 weeks ago. His scans have confirmed widespread liver, lymph node, and lung metastases. Alan has lost 10 kg in weight over 2 months and is awaiting results to assess eligibility for a clinical trial.

He remains upbeat, is convinced that he will "beat this cancer again" and is hopeful that the trial will provide the "magic drug" he needs. His wife is concerned that Alan is unwilling to accept his current predicament. They have never discussed prognosis with their oncologist. Yvonne is afraid of asking.

Alan has not completed the ACP provided by the community palliative care team. He has also not seen to any of his legal or financial affairs. Yvonne is understandably worried about the future.

Prior to commencing an ACP conversation, ensure you

- Understand your jurisdictions and organizational, legal, and governance procedures around ACP.
- Ensure you familiarize yourself with the documents and requirements for completion, witnessing, and record keeping.
- Check if your patient has completed an ACP, appointed a surrogate decision-maker before, and if there is a need or desire to update the ACP or revoke any appointments.

🔍 Key Point

In an initial ACP interaction, a clinician should

- Assess readiness for ACP by sensitively exploring a patient's desire for information about their disease, future treatment options, and prognosis.
- Present potential future clinical scenarios, treatment, or supportive care options. A cancer patient may not want to make specific decisions

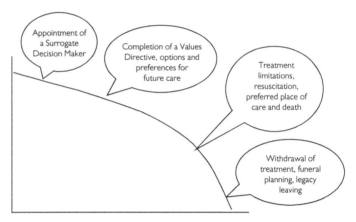

Figure 1.2 Advance Care Planning decision-making through the cancer trajectory.

about treatment limitations or end of life preferences at the early stages of their illness but may be willing to consider these options later (see Figure 1.2).

- Document any ACP discussion in a medical record and offer the opportunity to complete an ACP/Advance Directive or equivalent.

If a patient is deemed ready for ACP, the clinician may recommend that:

- The patient considers whom they may trust to appoint as their surrogate decision-maker if they lose the capacity to make decisions for themselves.
- The completion of a values statement or values directive is undertaken.
- Consideration of instructional directives that suggest parameters for treatment limitations, such as cardiopulmonary resuscitation, use of antibiotics, or admission into an intensive care unit. These decisions should be discussed with a trusted clinician.
- Consideration of other issues such as organ or tissue donation, prepared place of care and death, legacy leaving, and planning for a funeral.

An example of how an ACP conversation may be initiated is shown in Box 1.6 and an example of an ACP document is presented at the back of this book in Appendix 2.

What Are the Challenges of Completing an ACP in a Cancer Population?

ACP uptake in cancer patients remains poor, with only 15%–20% of patients completing written documentation.[19] Key barriers include:

- Discussions are timed inappropriately.
- Patients are waiting for their physicians to initiate the conversation.
- ACP conversations may be viewed as annihilating hope.
- Patients may choose to focus on the "now" rather than consider the future.
- ACP may evoke distress and anxiety.

Box 1.6 Example of How an ACP Conversation May Be Initiated

D: You mentioned to me that you are worried about what may occur in the future with regards to your illness. Is this something you would like to further discuss and plan for?

P: Yes, I am afraid to ask, but I think that it may be better to confront my fears. This is causing me and my wife much anxiety.

D: Well, yes. These conversations can be confronting. Many patients are anxious about taking about the future. However, many feel relieved after addressing their worries with a clinician they know and trust.

One approach to consider when we discuss your future is to have an advance care planning discussion. Have you heard of the term "advance care planning"?

P: Well, the nurse mentioned it and left me a form when she visited.

D: This is a conversation where we discuss your current illness and how it may change in the weeks and months ahead. Importantly, it is a conversation that addresses your values and the things that are important to you and your family, and how they may impact on how we make decisions with you. Importantly, it allows you to think about whom you may trust in your circle of family or friends to make decisions on your behalf if you cannot make them yourself. We will also discuss how you may like to be cared for when you get less well. Is this a conversation you would like to proceed with?

P: Yes, I think it would be helpful.

D: That's great. Let's make an appointment for you to come back to see me. In the meantime, here is some information for you to read about advance care planning. I suggest you read this with somebody you trust, such as the person you may want to appoint as your surrogate-decision maker and that you also invite them along when you return to see me. We can then address your questions and work through an Advance Care Planning document together.

Professional Issues and Service Implementation

Cultural Issues at the End of Life

What Is Culture, and Why Is It Important?

Due to increasing globalization and immigration in the last century, there have been profound worldwide demographic changes, with healthcare professionals increasingly caring for multicultural communities. Culture is one of several social constructs used to signify diversity among individuals and groups.

Culture can be defined as a body of values, perspectives, beliefs, behaviors, and traditions salient within a specific group of people and encompasses language, dress, customs, food, societal structures, art, and religious characteristics.

The differences in the cultural beliefs, valtues, and healthcare practices of diverse communities are particularly relevan at the end of life, with the need for culturally sensitive and competent cross-cultural communication.[20] Cultural differences can influence health-related decision-making and lead to several ethical dilemmas when care is only provided through a Western clinical and ethical framework.

Individualizing Care for Diverse Communities

While cultural specifics may be broadly applicable to people from similar cultural backgrounds, clinicians need to recognize that no cultural group is homogeneous, with beliefs varying even within families, sometimes across generations. As such, one of the initial steps of the clinician–patient interaction is often inquiring about the individual patient's cultural background to understand each patient's view of their situation, their expectations for how to make decisions, who will be involved, and what type of care will follow. For diverse communities, cultural considerations can include, but are not limited to:

- Preferred language used
- Attitudes to healthcare, including:
  - Role of healthcare professionals
  - Concepts of disease, including terminology used
  - Disclosure of diagnosis and prognosis
  - Medical treatments including opioid drugs, sedatives, hydration, and nutrition
  - Ways of conceptualizing death and dying
- Approach to decision-making and communication:
  - Individualism versus collectivism
  - Differences in the interpretation of nonverbal communication and indirect communication
  - Low levels of literacy
- Role of the family unit:
  - How a family is defined
  - Provision of care, including gender roles and care of the elderly
  - Involvement in health-related decision-making
- The preferred setting of care:
  - In some cultures, there may be a strong desire to remain at home and resistance to institutionalized care.
- Diet and food choices
- Personal care rituals and privacy issues
- Customs surrounding death, burial, cremation, and bereavement

Communication, Cultural Expectations, and Role of the Family

Therapeutic communication between clinicians and patients of diverse cultural backgrounds can be challenging and may relate to issues as listed in Table 1.5. This conflict in cultural expectations and resultant dilemmas of patient autonomy, patient-centered versus family-centered decision-making, truth-telling, information withholding, and collusion with the family unit can

Table 1.5 Issues to be Considered in Cross-Cultural Communication

Use of specific terminology such as "cancer" or "palliative care"	Belief that discussing these topics may bring about death and that the timing of death can only be determined by God.
Language and the use of interpreters	Family care-givers from culturally diverse backgrounds often assist with interpretation during consultations. A professional interpreter is preferred due to greater accuracy in conveying information to patients and to ensure the veracity of information that is conveyed when interpreting.
Expectations surrounding disclosure of disease and prognosis	The family unit may request withholding of information and to have initial conversations away from the patient. Patients may be provided with vague, indirect, nuanced information with the intent of protecting the terminally ill patient from emotional distress and loss of hope.
Autonomy may not be the preeminent precept	Family-centric decision-making may be prioritized over individual patient autonomy. Decision-making may be completely relinquished to health professionals, who may be viewed with significant authority, and reflect the family's preference for a directive approach to decision-making.

be challenging to address.[21] It is important to remember that each individual patient has a right to choose to be told or not told their diagnosis and participate in conversations surrounding their ongoing care. If a patient wants to participate in these conversations, a strategy to minimize conflict involves organizing a doctor–patient consultation with the family unit and a professional interpreter present. This enables the family to hear the patient's request for information, including the breadth of information they would like and subsequent information relayed firsthand.

Ethical and Legal Issues at the End of Life

Communicating the nuances of common ethical and legal issues can be challenging at the end of life. It requires:

• An understanding of the jurisdictional law, professional guidance, and evidence pertaining to a particular issue
• The application of a considered ethical framework for decision-making
• An appreciation of cultural and individual nuances
• Confirmation of patient capacity and an understanding of their beliefs and preferences
• An appreciation of the patient's clinical condition and outlook

The following are the commonly faced ethical and legal issues:

- Exploring decision-making capacity, advanced directives and surrogate decision-making:
  - Capacity may be affected in a deteriorating patient due to delirium, drowsiness, loss of cognitive processing, and executive decision-making impairment due to disease and aging.
  - Referring to a previously completed advanced directive or identifying the appointed surrogate decision maker
- Withdrawal or assisted hydration and nutrition:
  - The provision of food and drink are essential to human flourishing, but when provided in a clinically assisted setting, they are classed as treatment rather than basic care. Communication requires sensitivity, an understanding of commonly held misconceptions and the ability to negotiate acceptable outcomes. For instance, a family may accept the discontinuation of nasogastric feeding if oral risk feeding is allowed.
- Cardiopulmonary resuscitation:
  - Discussions around cardiopulmonary resuscitation require imparting information on poor outcomes and impaired quality of life with survival.
  - Conversations for appropriate patients with advanced illness should include more appropriate treatment options that could be offered, such as transfer to a high dependency unit or acute hospital.
- Euthanasia and physician-assisted suicide:
  - Terms vary across jurisdictions. Euthanasia/Physician Assisted Suicide (Europe), Medical Aid in Dying (Canada) and Voluntary Assisted Dying (Australia) describe the act of administrating medication (patient or clinician administered) in accordance with the steps and process set out in law where such legislation is passed.
  - Increasingly the above is viewed as an acceptable mode of dying, with patients wanting to determine their time, manner, and place of death. Palliative care services in many countries try to avoid involvement with E-PAS processes while optimally palliating symptoms during this time. Thus, the ethical principle of non-abandonment is upheld alongside a professional's conscientious objection to a process they disagree with.
  - Communication requires the ability to explore such a desire in an open and nonjudgmental manner, ensuring that critical issues such as depression, demoralization, and existential distress are appropriately addressed.

Examples of common errors in communication and the more appropriate approach are highlighted in Table 1.6.

Training and Service Development Issues

Early integration of palliative care with standard oncological care is now well established, meeting the psychological and physical needs of cancer patients.[22] Introduction to palliative care and end of life topics are best initiated by the treating oncologist or clinician though such conversations continue to occur too late and often at a point of crisis. In order to achieve excellence in end of life care, cancer clinicians require training to achieve the core competencies of skills, knowledge, experience, attributes, and behaviors.[23] The core categories that may be addressed for skill development are summarized in Box 1.7.

Table 1.6 Common Errors of Communication of Ethical and Legal Issues

Ethical or Legal Issue Communicated	Common Communication Style	Perception of Patient and Family	Preferred Communication Style
Withholding or withdrawing treatment	"We will be discontinuing antibiotics and fluid today as it is futile treatment."	There is nothing more that the medical team are going to do, precipitating feelings of abandonment.	"At this point, providing intravenous fluids and antibiotics may be causing more harm than benefit. We are going to manage thirst using mouth care, and her cough with the use of medications and physiotherapy."
Cardiopulmonary resuscitation	"We will be enacting a Do-Not-Resuscitate order in your medical records"	The doctors are giving up, discontinuing all my treatment, and will simply let me die	"If your heart stops beating on its own, we will not commence chest compressions which may cause you significant harm and distress. We will instead ensure you remain comfortable and provided with all the necessary medications and care"

Internationally, the challenge remains as to how services in resource-constrained settings implement palliative care when most guidelines are based on research conducted in maximal resource institutions. The American Society of Clinical Oncology resource-stratified guidelines[24] provide expert guidance to clinicians and policymakers on implementing palliative care of patients with cancer and their caregivers in resource-constrained settings. The guidelines recommend that healthcare providers and healthcare system decision makers should be guided by the recommendations for the highest stratum of resources available, with guidelines intended to complement, and not replace, local guidelines. Services are stratified to: General, Basic (Primary Health Care), Limited (District), Enhanced (Regional) and Maximal (National), with recommendations made of the following:

1. Palliative care models
2. Timing for involvement of palliative care
3. Workforce, knowledge, and skills
4. Nurse role in pain management
5. Spiritual care
6. Social work/counseling
7. Opioid availability

Box 1.7 Core Categories for Skill Development for Excellence in End of Life Care

- Communication skills that integrate palliative care
  - The development of a range of sensitive and facilitative communication skills,[29] e.g., (1) What is happening?, (2) How do you (and I) feel?, and (3) What is important?
  - Utilize a coherent strategy when making urgent medical decisions, e.g., REMAP (**R**eframe the situation; **E**xpect emotion and acknowledge it; **M**ap out important values; **A**lign with your patient and their family; **P**lan treatments to match values)
- Psychosocial skills
  - An ability to anticipate and diagnose commonly occurring issues such as depression, despair, loss of hope, and poor patient and family understanding of illness and treatment
- Symptom management skills
  - Management of basic pain and other symptoms, and palliative care emergencies appropriately
- Teamwork skills
  - A collaborative approach to managing care with other members of a multidisciplinary team
- Interpersonal skills
  - The ability to recognize and understand personal reactions that may occur when working with the dying and bereaved. An appreciation of emotional vulnerability, compassion fatigue, burnout, and when to seek available supports

References

1. Mazor KM, Beard RL, Alexander GL, et al. Patients' and family members' views on patient-centered communication during cancer care. Psycho-Oncology. 2013;22(11):2487–2495. https://doi.org/10.1002/pon.3317.

2. Gilligan T, Coyle N, Frankel RM, et al. Patient–clinician communication: American Society of Clinical Oncology consensus guideline. J Clin Oncol. 2017;35(31):3618–3632. https://doi.org/10.1200/JCO.2017.75.2311.

3. Maex E, De Valck C. Key elements of communication in cancer care. In Stiefel F, Editor. Communication in Cancer Care. Berlin, Heidelberg: Springer-Verlag Berlin Heidelberg; 2006. Pages 11–15.

4. Pichler T, Rohrmoser A, Letsch A, et al. Information, communication, and cancer patients' trust in the physician: What challenges do we have to face in an era of precision cancer medicine? Support Care Cancer. 2021;29(4):2171–2178. https://doi.org/10.1007/s00520-020-05692-7.

5. Keinki C, Momberg A, Clauß K, et al. Effect of question prompt lists for cancer patients on communication and mental health outcomes: A systematic review. Patient Educ Couns. 2021;104(6):1335–1346. https://doi.org/10.1016/j.pec.2021.01.012.

6. Clayton J, Butow P, Tattersall M, et al. Asking questions can help: Development and preliminary evaluation of a question prompt list for palliative care patients. Br J Cancer. 2003;89(11):2069–2077. https://doi.org/10.1038/sj.bjc.6601380.

7. Rieger KL, Hack TF, Beaver K, Schofield P. Should consultation recording use be a practice standard? A systematic review of the effectiveness and implementation of consultation recordings. Psycho-Oncology. 2018;27(4):1121–1128. https://doi.org/10.1002/pon.4592.

8. Berg MN, Ngune I, Schofield P, et al. Effectiveness of online communication skills training for cancer and palliative care health professionals: A systematic review. Psycho-Oncology. 2021;30(9):1405–1419. https://doi.org/10.1002/pon.5702.

9. Bylund CL, Brown RF, Bialer PA, Levin TT, Lubrano di Ciccone B, Kissane DW. Developing and implementing an advanced communication training program in oncology at a comprehensive cancer center. J Cancer Educ. 2011;26(4):604–611. https://doi.org/ 10.1007/s13187-011-0226-y.

10. von Blankenburg P, Hoff M, Rief W, et al. Assessing patients' preferences for breaking bad news according to the SPIKES-Protocol: The MABBAN scale. Patient Edu Couns. 2020;103(8):1623–1629. https://doi.org/10.1016/j.pec.2020.02.036.

11. Hui D. Prognostication of survival in patients with advanced cancer: Predicting the unpredictable? Cancer Control. 2015;22(4):489–497. https://doi.org/ 10.1177/107327481502200415

12. Christakis NA, Lamont EB. Extent and determinants of error in doctors' prognoses in terminally ill patients: Prospective cohort study. BMJ. 2000;320(7233):469–472. https://doi.org/10.1136/bmj.320.7233.469.

13. Hui d, Ross J Park M, et al. Predicting survival in patients with advanced cancer in the last weeks of life: How accurate are prognostic models compared to clinicians' estimates? Palliat Med. 2020;34(1):126–133. https://doi.org/ 10.1177/0269216319873261.

14. Breitbart W, Rosenfeld B, Pessin H, et al. Meaning-centered group psychotherapy: An effective intervention for improving psychological well-being in patients with advanced cancer. J Clin Oncol. 2015;33(7):749–754. https://doi.org/10.1200/JCO.2014.57.2198.

15. Phelps AC, Lauderdale KE, Alcorn S, et al. Addressing spirituality within the care of patients at the end of life: Perspectives of patients with advanced cancer, oncologists, and oncology nurses. J Clin Oncol. 2012;30(20):2538–2544. https://doi.org/10.1200/JCO.011.40.3766.

16. Möllerberg ML, Årestedt K, Swahnberg K, et al. Family sense of coherence and its associations with hope, anxiety and symptoms of depression in persons with cancer in palliative phase and their family members: A cross-sectional study. Palliat Med. 2019;33(10):1310–1318. https://doi.org/10.1177/02692 16319866653.

17. Coyle N, Kissane DW. Conducting a family meeting. In Handbook of Communication in Oncology and Palliative Care. Oxford: Oxford University Press; 2017. Pages: 165–175.

18. Sudore RL, Lum HD, You JJ, et al. Defining advance care planning for adults: A consensus definition from a multidisciplinary Delphi panel. J Pain Symptom Manage. 2017;53(5):821–832.e1. https://doi.org/10.1016/j.jpainsymman.2016.12.331.

19. Bestvina CM, Polite BN. Implementation of advance care planning in oncology: A review of the literature. J Oncol Pract. 2017;13(10):657–662. https://doi.org/10.1200/JOP.2017.021246.

20. Cain CL, Surbone A, Elk R, et al. Culture and palliative care: Preferences, communication, meaning, and mutual decision making. J Pain Symptom Manage. 2018;55(5):1408–1419. https://doi.org/10.1016/j.jpainsymman.2018.01.007.

21. Grassi L. Communicating anticancer treatment cessation and transition to palliative care: The need for a comprehensive and culturally relevant, person-centered approach. Cancer. 2015;121(23):4104–4107. https://doi.org/10.1002/cncr.29638.

22. Ferrell BR, Temel JS, Temin S, et al. Integration of palliative care into standard oncology care: American Society of Clinical Oncology clinical practice guideline update. J Clin Oncol. 2017;35(1):96–112. https://doi.org/ 10.1200/JCO.2016.70.1474.

23. Back A, Friedman T, Abrahm J. Palliative care skills and new resources for oncology practices: Meeting the palliative care needs of patients with cancer and their families. Am Soc Clin Oncol Educ Book. 2020;40:1–9. https://doi.org/10.1200/EDBK_100022.

24. Osman H, Shrestha S, Temin S, et al. Palliative care in the global setting: ASCO resource-stratified practice guideline. J Glob Oncol. 2018;4:1–24. https://doi.org/10.1200/JGO.18.00026.

Further Reading

Kissane DW, Bultz BD, Butow PN, Bylund CL, Noble S, Wilkinson S, Editors. Oxford Textbook of Communication in Oncology and Palliative Care. 2nd ed. (65 chapters, 434 pages). Oxford: Oxford University Press; 2017. This is a comprehensive reference book to guide communication skills training and it provides myriad examples of communication strategies in the palliative care setting authored by many of the world's leading academics.

Stiefel F, Editor. Communication in Cancer Care (12 chapters, 125 pages). Berlin Heidelberg, Berlin, Heidelberg: Springer; 2006. This short book examines in depth some of the particularly complex areas of communication in cancer care. The authors represent a variety of disciplines, providing a multiperspective and international summary of issues.

Surbone A, Zwitter M, Rajer M, Stiefel R, Editors. New Challenges in Communication with Cancer Patients (42 chapters, 504 pages). New York: Springer US; 2013. This book focuses on some of the more recent challenges faced by cancer clinicians internationally. Its chapters on communication in hereditary cancers, children, and psychological challenges faced by the practitioner are welcomed.

Angelos P, Editor. Ethical Issues in Cancer Patient Care (10 chapters, 149 pages). New York: Springer US; 2000. This short yet comprehensive book addresses some of the key ethical issues related to communication, cross-cultural care, and religious and spiritual concerns in the cancer patient.

Elwyn, G, Edwards A, Thompson R, Editors. Shared Decision Making in Health Care. Achieving Evidence-Based Patient Choice (45 chapters, 336 pages). Oxford: Oxford University Press; 2016. The concise chapters in the book provide current evidence on how shared decision-making promotes a clinician-centered approach to care with a focus on translation of topics covered into practice.

Chapter 2

Anxiety Disorders

Daniel McFarland, William Pirl, and Maggie Watson

Learning Objectives

After reading this chapter, the clinician will be able to:

1. Describe formal anxiety disorders in cancer patients receiving palliative and end of life care.
2. Outline key investigations and tools for the assessment and diagnosis of anxiety disorders.
3. Make an informed differential diagnosis considering medical and psychological causes of anxiety at the end of life.
4. Implement clinical management options to address anxiety disorders.
5. Understand relevant professional, ethical, and cultural issues for managing anxiety disorders in patients with advanced cancer and at the end of life.

Background Evidence

Prevalence

Anxiety disorders are common in cancer patients or family caregivers at the end of life and are likely to complicate supportive care. Anxiety symptoms are reported in up to 50% of patients with cancer, but diagnostic, interview-based primary anxiety disorders have much lower prevalence of 10.3% in cancer and palliative care settings according to a meta-analysis of 94 studies.[1] This meta-analysis also found that 38.2% of patients had at least one diagnoseable interview-based mood disorder, with 19.4% classified as adjustment disorder (see Chapter 3). Interview-based anxiety and depressive disorders were highly comorbid and associated with each other.

In patients with advanced cancer initializing inpatient palliative care, 47% of family caregivers report significant anxiety on the Generalized Anxiety Disorder-7 (GAD-7). compared to 11.5% of family caregivers of breast cancer patients receiving outpatient oncologic treatment. [2,3]

Theoretical Models

Anxiety in advanced cancer patients can be categorized as follows:

1. psychological reaction to the experience of illness;
2. primary anxiety disorder;

3. anxiety symptoms comorbid with other nonanxiety mood disorders (e.g., depression) precipitated or exacerbated by cancer and related events;
4. existential, death anxiety.

Sources of anxiety in the advanced cancer setting are ubiquitous. Anxiety can be related directly to the state of illness. For example, anxiety arises when patients are dyspneic from hypoxia (lack of oxygen) in advanced lung cancer, or metastatic sarcoma involving the lungs, metabolic states requiring heightened respiration to alleviate hypercarbia (e.g., sepsis), cardiac dysfunction (e.g., arrhythmias), or pulmonary circulation shunting resulting from pulmonary disease (e.g., restrictive and reactive airway diseases, collapsed or trapped lung, atelectasis, etc.).

Alternatively, anxiety may be the result of cancer treatments and supportive medications (e.g., corticosteroids to prevent chemotherapy-induced nausea). Substance use, abuse, and withdrawal can also be a source of anxiety. Although anxiety is pervasive throughout the cancer trajectory, the palliative setting and advancing disease states frequently engender increasing anxiety as a reaction to stress.

Specific categories of anxiety disorder include:
- generalized anxiety disorder
- panic disorder
- phobias
- posttraumatic stress disorder
- pathological fear of dying (i.e., death anxiety)

Lung, gynecologic, and hematologic cancers often confer the highest rates of anxiety.[4] In addition, later stage at diagnosis or progressive disease trajectory (e.g., recurrence, advanced disease, or advancing illness), and concomitant symptom burden (e.g., pain, insomnia, breathlessness), are associated with more anxiety disorders and anxiety symptoms. Factors associated with the precipitation of anxiety are exceedingly important for the psycho-oncologist to understand since they are associated with recalcitrant anxiety and other psychiatric symptoms. For example, it may be difficult to adequately treat anxiety symptoms that are associated with unremitting pain or other uncontrolled physical symptoms. Physical symptoms such as dyspnea, pain, gastrointestinal dysfunction, nausea, vomiting, anorexia, declining physical states, poor executive function, and even recalcitrant hiccups are associated with anxiety and make its treatment more difficult. Underlying reasons for anxiety should be addressed along with the symptomatic relief from anxiety.

Death Anxiety

At the end of life, death anxiety has been described in 32% of patients with at least moderate severity.[5] Addressing death anxiety is a uniquely challenging endeavor given the inherent uselessness of reassurance. Therefore, careful assessment is needed because patients may not always disclose the source of their anxiety and a patient-specific, tailored approach is needed. Patients have very specific worries from practical issues to existential dread. These should be explored on their own terms.

Fear of Cancer Progression

Fear of cancer progression (FCP) may occur in patients with controlled metastatic disease and present with spikes of anxiety occurring around the time of surveillance imaging or laboratory testing of tumor markers. This type of anxiety has been given the colloquial terms, *scanitis* or *markeritis*. Patients may become severely anxious before or during tests, preoccupied with minute changes and dwell on the meaning of results to the point that quality of life is significantly disrupted.

Consequences of Anxiety

Anxiety at end of life may interfere with the ability to comprehend and engage in disease-related decision making, adherence with recommended treatments, actual response to treatments, the efficacy of addressing other symptoms (e.g., pain), and undermine coping mechanisms. Intermittent or pervasive anxiety may undermine clear thought processes and prevent patients from making decisions most consistent with their values and wishes. Most immediately, this may come in the form of medication nonadherence, trouble maintaining social support systems, difficulty keeping medical appointments and keeping up with activities of daily living. Functional impairment may also be ascertained by assessing health-related quality of life (HRQOL). Longitudinal assessment of anxiety is an important indicator of severity but some types of anxiety, like panic or posttraumatic stress disorders, carry burden even when patients are not having active symptoms. Patients may be using techniques such as avoidance, compulsions, or other behavior mechanisms to avert symptoms. Thus, pathological anxiety leads to life interference and functional impairment as it applies to the patient's approach to medical care and maintaining relationships and social supports.

Pathophysiology

Although psychiatric disorders are increasingly understood in biological terms, the etiology and pathophysiology of most anxiety disorders continues to be questioned.[6] The general stress response is useful in understanding anxiety symptoms. Stress responses are regulated by feedback mechanisms related to hypothalamic-pituitary-adrenal (HPA) axis activation, which begins with corticotrophin-releasing factor (CRF) synthesis and secretion and leads to glucocorticoid production. In the cancer context, peripheral inflammation is generally increased due to cancer-related tissue damage, immune activation, and cancer treatments. Excessive inflammation has been shown to decrease negative feedback responsiveness to glucocorticoids, creating unregulated stress responses and contributing to increased anxiety symptoms in patients with cancer.[7]

Another biologically driven mechanism of cancer-related anxiety is the down regulation of γ-aminobutyric acid (GABA), the most prominent inhibitory neurotransmitter that is an active target of anxiolytic medications. Downregulation of GABA allows for increased excitatory neurologic activity associated with stress, anxiety, and related behavioral changes. The noradrenergic, cholinergic, and dopaminergic systems are also responsible for the production and regulation of anxiety. Genetic and hereditary factors are associated with anxiety disorder, the production of anxiety symptoms, and anxiety treatment responses.

Presenting Problems

Key Symptoms and Signs

Symptoms are experienced by the patient while signs are seen by clinicians and others. Although signs and symptoms are frequently concordant, patients may not be aware of what they are experiencing internally or perceive how their behaviors or actions are seen externally while under the pressures of cancer. Patients may not be aware of how they are feeling, especially immediately after learning about cancer recurrence. If this continues after an initial period of shock, it could be the result of *alexithymia*, or the inability to identify felt emotion. Acutely, patients may experience bodily temperature fluctuations, cold sweats, palpitations, nausea and vomiting, diarrhea, constipation, heartburn, and other gastrointestinal symptoms. Chronically, patients develop fatigue and exhaustion in addition to feeling depleted, overwhelmed, and lack a sense of self efficacy.

Although self-report measures frequently uncover anxiety that otherwise would have been left undiscussed, the clinician's intuition and observation may and should guide the diagnosis.

It is important to evaluate for "red flags," although a wide range of expected or normative reactions should be anticipated. Pathological responses and anxiety may be detected in what is *not said or acknowledged* just as much as in the manifest content. Worrisome, "red flags" of anxiety disorders and their consequences include; social withdrawal, loss of executive functioning, preoccupation with mortality and other morbid outcomes.

Individual pathological responses may be discovered when patients share responses to past stressors and allow for the addition of collateral sources of information. Interestingly, there is an arc of psychological adjustment where symptoms may peak and abate as the patient adjusts to new information. Clinicians should look out for longitudinal patterns of anxiety symptoms that do not reflect psychological adjustment as these more likely indicate clinically significant anxiety. Table 2.1 highlights important aspects of the psychological and physical components of anxiety disorders and symptoms.

While physical manifestations of anxiety, especially in a constellation and without underlying causative medical factors, are highly suggestive of anxiety disorders, the cognitive components are more highly diagnostic of anxiety disorders in many respects. The clinician needs to assess both thought processes and content.

The patient may not report somatic symptoms but may have free-flowing anxious thoughts about multiple topics and express an inability to turn away from these thoughts.

Table 2.1 Signs and Symptoms of Anxiety

Psychological	• Worry, apprehension, fear, and sadness.
	• Patient may be able to identify focus or source of these symptoms.
	• Often nonspecific and "free-floating"
	• Crying spells, ruminations
	• Typical complaint (especially at night): inability to "turn off" one's thoughts
	• Death anxiety
Physical	• Tachycardia and tachypnea
	• Tremor, diaphoresis, nausea, dry mouth, insomnia, and anorexia
	• Poor physical symptom control (intractable, medical refractoriness)
Timing- intermittent: relapse and remitting, Increasing/decreasing over hours or days	• In response to a stressor (e.g., anticipation of pending diagnostic testing or procedures) with resolution if/when the stressor passes.
Timing- persistent: symptoms persist throughout the day and are pervasive	• Typical of primary anxiety disorders. • Comorbid depressive disorders. • Reactions to chronic stressors (e.g., fear of cancer recurrence, family/financial problems). • Side effects of regularly prescribed medications.
Timing- paroxysmal: characteristic of panic attacks	• Severe palpitations, diaphoresis, and nausea. There is often a sense of great fear of a catastrophic event, described as a "Feeling of impending doom" • Usually lasts for at least several minutes. The frequency is variable, with multiple possible events in a single day

The following questions are helpful:
• "Have you worried persistently beyond what you would expect?"
• "Have your worries caused you to be concerned?"
• "Can you distract yourself from worry for a period of time?"

This would be most consistent with generalized anxiety disorders (GADs) or fear of recurring panic attacks with a clear description and feelings about the first recognized panic attack is diagnostic for panic disorder. For patients with panic disorder especially, timing of physical and emotional symptoms is key. Symptoms are typically described as severe but lasting only a few minutes. They may recur inconsistently or up to several times per day. Commonly associated physical symptoms are; severe heart palpitations (e.g., "my heart feels like it's coming out of my chest"), diaphoresis, and nausea accompanied by an impending sense of "doom." Preoccupation with consequences of disease, treatment, cancer progression, or death is common. But for patients with death anxiety or FCP these concerns will interfere with daily functioning and tasks, relationships, and the patient's quality of life.

While anxiety can have physical components, these can sometimes overlap with symptoms from underlying medical issues. For example, the sudden onset of panic in an older individual with cancer and no prior history of panic disorder is suggestive of a pulmonary embolism, which creates a sudden depletion of oxygen and is relatively common in cancer settings. Pulmonary emboli precipitate panic and should be ruled out in patients with risk factors and sudden onset anxiety. Anxiety is always a diagnosis of exclusion and careful attention must be given to the physical symptoms and their context.

⚲ Key Points

- Patients with concurrent depression, other known anxiety disorders or substance abuse, high symptom burden, low social supports, or progressive cancer are more likely to have anxiety symptoms.
- Medications such as steroids or beta agonists (e.g., albuterol) can induce anxiety symptoms.
- Cancer-specific agents can cause anxiety either by direct neurotoxicity (e.g., high dose cytarabine) or via thyroid dysfunction (e.g., small molecule tyrosine kinase inhibitors can be thyrotoxic leading to hyperthyroidism, followed by hypothyroidism or other chronic thyroid abnormalities).
- Patients who overuse, or abuse stimulants (e.g., caffeine, methyl phenidate, cocaine) may present with anxiety related to these substances.
- Patients who are tolerant to benzodiazepines or withdrawing from nervous system depressants such as alcohol or opiates frequently have significant anxiety symptoms. The pharmacological management of alcohol withdrawal in patients at the end of life should be the institution of benzodiazepines with an exceedingly gradual taper that does not precipitate anxiety.

⚲ Key Problems

- **Overlapping symptoms**: Anxiety has cognitive and somatic components that demonstrate significant interactions and coupling effects. Anxiety leads to uncomfortable bodily tension, which can progress to pervasive fatigue and a feeling of bodily exhaustion.
- **Nonrecognition**: Anxiety symptoms in the setting of cancer are frequently normalized by non-mental-health clinicians. For this reason, and perhaps others, it is frequently difficult for non-mental-health professionals to diagnose mental health disorders such as anxiety, even with the help of clinical screening.[8] Unfortunately, implementing screening does not solve the problem of nonrecognition, since screening tools capture nondiagnostic symptoms of distress or anxiety and have much greater sensitivity than specificity.

⚲ Key Point

Screening is not a perfect solution and a clinical diagnostic interview is still necessary to diagnose anxiety disorders in patients at the end of life and to understand the root causes and implications of anxiety disorders and symptoms.

Contributory Physical Disease Factors

The correlation between physical symptom burden and mood symptoms is exceedingly strong. The raw number of symptoms is associated with greater anxiety and depression, which is particularly relevant for patients at the end of life.[9] Reduced mobility or inability to participate in activities of daily living (ADLs) is strikingly anxiety-producing for many patients who are reaching the end of life.

🔍 Key Physical Symptoms

Certain physical symptoms predict higher rates of anxiety. These include breathlessness, heart palpitations, gastrointestinal symptoms, chronic or persistent pain, and migraine headaches, which are closely associated with the development of anxiety. For example, pulmonary embolism (e.g., blood clot that lodges in the lungs) can cause sudden reduction in blood oxygen levels (i.e., hypoxemia), pain, and enhanced sympathetic nervous system activity (e.g., noradrenergic) and precipitate anxiety. Cancer, advanced age, and other medical comorbidities lead to clotting or thrombus production. Therefore, pulmonary emboli are very common in palliative or end of life situations. At the same time, it should be noted that even minor appearing symptoms can become highly distressing, especially when they become chronically present, and prevent important activities (e.g., leaving home and needing to use the restroom, or being afraid to eat in public, etc.). A prime example of how a minor appearing symptom can cause significant distress is with "hiccups" as they can become persistent, uncomfortable, distressing, and worsen quality of life.

Also note the following:

- **Akathisia**: The inner restlessness occurring as a side-effect of antinausea or neuroleptic medications is easily missed.
- **Medication tolerance**: Rebound anxiety with the habitual use of benzodiazepines is very common, causing insomnia, physical restlessness, and bodily discomfort. Also, cessation of dopamine blocking agents used to prevent and treat nausea (e.g., prochlorperazine, olanzapine) may precipitate anxiety.

In terms of treatment, there is a general concordance that reducing physical symptoms tends to reduce anxiety, and treating anxiety reduces physical symptom severity.

Agitation/Delirium

Patients with advanced cancer and other advanced diseases experience delirium and even agitation (see Chapter 5). At the end of life, most patients (88%) experience delirium and cognitive impairment.[10] The experience of delirium is highly anxiety producing because mental faculties, ability to rationalize, and understand the world are compromised. Patients have various levels of insight. Once the period of delirium has passed, they say almost unanimously that the experience was terrifying.

Key Points

- Patients who are delirious or encephalopathic seem to lose periods of time and then regain awareness, highlighting the waxing and waning hallmark of delirium.
- Disordered thought processes and disinhibition may lead to agitation and even violence that the patient may later regret.
- Patients who are delirious experience anxiety while delirious and from the repercussions of delirium.
- An array of medication withdrawal can precipitate delirium and anxiety (e.g., narcotic, benzodiazepines, anticholinergic medications). An attempt to limit many of these medications is common at the end of life in an attempt to reduce side effects.

The temporality of symptom development is very important for understanding their relationship and how to address with psychopharmacology. In the setting of delirium, it is important to address delirium first, investigating for its cause and treating such etiology.

NOTE: Antipsychotic medications can restore the sleep-wake cycle, ameliorate delirium and/or behavioral outbursts, in addition to relieving anxiety. Anxiety that is particularly severe can cause psychosis and cognitive dysfunction as the patient appears behaviorally dysfunctional. In this setting, the anxiety would have come first and attempts at treating the anxiety with benzodiazepines in addition to anti-psychotic medications would be indicated.

Assessment and Differential Diagnosis

Patients who present with mood symptoms should receive a comprehensive assessment for a broad range of anxiety-related diagnoses. Given the overlap with other affective disorders, it is imperative that primary anxiety disorders are distinguished from other mood disorders (i.e., depressive disorders, see Chapter 4) with anxiety symptoms. At the same time, the etiology of anxiety symptoms in cancer and other medical settings is extensive. Not only does anxiety spring from psychological stressors and baseline personality characteristics but also underlying physiology, altered hormone functioning (e.g., hyperthyroidism), physical symptoms (tachycardia, dyspnea), direct cancer involvement (e.g., primary brain tumor or metastases), or medication side effects (e.g., beta agonist inhalers, steroids, excessive thyroid replacement, encephalopathy from cyclophosphamide or other chemotherapy, renal or other organ dysfunction), or stopping medication or chemical substances (e.g., alcohol, benzodiazepines, tobacco, or stopping other anxiolytics or anxiolytic-like medications like baclofen).

In patients with complex medical issues, it is imperative to consider anxiety due to another medical condition and substance/medication-induced anxiety disorder. This will require history taking in addition to laboratory assessment. History should alert the clinician to underlying concomitant illness, medications, and the presence of additional symptoms or anxiety symptoms. The history should focus on the timing of symptoms, level of wakefulness, and assess for any periods of confusion, which would be altered in patients with anxious delirium. It is recommended that:

- Vital signs should be reviewed longitudinally for the presence of hypoxia, tachycardia, and tachypnea, for example.
- Do not overlook serotonin syndrome (fever, flushing, hypertension, and hyperreflexia) due to drug interactions with opioids, antiemetics, or antibiotics.
- In addition, laboratory assessment should be sent for thyroid function and to rule out hyperthyroidism specifically.
- Laboratory assessment of liver function may also indicate ongoing alcohol use or abuse, nutritional status, and other electrolyte abnormalities associated with mental status changes (hyper/hypocalemia, lactatemia, hyper/hyponatremia).

Evaluation of renal function will suggest how well the patient may be metabolizing other medications that could lead to anxiety. Those medications might be steroids, beta-agonists, caffeine and other stimulants, or toxicity from cytotoxic drugs, antibiotics, or other medications.

Other major categories of anxiety disorders should be considered such as trauma and stressor-related disorders (posttraumatic stress disorder), specific phobia (e.g., blood draws), social anxiety, GAD, panic disorder, and obsessive compulsive disorder (OCD) and related disorders. Working through this differential diagnosis requires history taking and collateral information and sometimes observation over the course of treatment or hospitalization. These diagnoses are not mutually exclusive and should also be evaluated with concurrent non-anxiety-related disorders in mind.

🔍 Key Point

Most importantly, depression and demoralization are highly comorbid with anxiety symptoms and should be thoroughly and repeatedly assessed.

Other affective disorders such as bipolar disorder and other psychotic disorders should be considered especially for a patient demonstrating odd

---

Box 2.1 Laboratory Tests to Evaluate Anxiety States

1. Electrolytes, urea, and creatinine
2. Thyroid function tests (TSH, free T4)
3. Liver function tests (serum bilirubin, albumin, clotting factors) and enzyme tests (alkaline phosphatase [ALP], alanine transaminase [ALT], aspartate aminotransferase [AST], gamma-glutamyl transpeptidase [GGT])
4. Calcium, MAGNESIUM
5. Consider electrocardiogram
6. Full blood examination for anaemia

Further Tests in Recalcitrant States

7. Tests of pheochromocytoma
8. Paraneoplastic panel (anti-hu, ra, ma)

Box 2.2 Safety Assessments

Should be made routinely and as needed in all patients regardless of anxiety symptoms. Agitation, anxiety, along with impulsivity, a recent loss, and a terminal illness *are all risk factors for suicide*, which is generally about twice as common in patients with cancer.

beliefs or internal preoccupation. Somatic symptoms and related disorders should be considered in patients with illness or bodily preoccupation. The cancer setting may require addressing existential concerns and the nature of the relationship between the patient and his or her oncology providers.

It is imperative to maintain a broad working differential diagnosis of anxiety when assessing patients with cancer, since anxiety is not always related to cancer or may be only peripherally. That is, common assumptions about why patients are having anxiety may be wrong. The significant life event of cancer is superimposed on patients' lives, which may have been or become psychosocially complicated prior to the diagnosis.

Certain timepoints are known to induce suicidal behavior multifold above the general population.[11] Suicide risk appears to be highest after diagnosis or recurrence but also increases with increasing symptom burden and advanced disease.

Clinical assessments should start with listening for a judicious period time to assess thought process and thought content. Listening will also provide information about the patient's insight and judgment. Scales and questionnaires that assess anxiety provide rich data that can be followed reliably over time. A sense of collaboration may be established for clinicians and patients who discuss the scale results in real time. Scales can help clinicians answer the essential clinical question regarding anxiety: How much is too much? Everyone experiences nervousness since it is an adaptive part of living and an essential emotion experienced throughout the life cycle. It signals danger and motivates action or change. But pathological anxiety is paralyzing, which can cause significant decrements in HRQOL and adversely affect cancer-related treatments (e.g., adherence, treatment decisions, support system/relationships, related psychosomatic symptoms such as pain, insomnia, fatigue). Accurate identification and assessment of anxiety can improve EOL and palliative experiences for patients with cancer.

Scales to Assess Anxiety

Scales can be used to screen for general or specific psychological symptoms such as anxiety in patients with cancer. Scales are also useful to monitor symptoms longitudinally in a consistent manner. Scales are used in research studies and clinical care; they help strengthen diagnostic acumen and personalize clinical care. Self-report measures do not lessen the need for clinical interviews but may make interviews more targeted.

- **Generalized Anxiety Disorder-7 (GAD-7)**

    Anxiety in cancer settings is commonly measured using the GAD-7. This brief seven item measure was meant to evaluate generalized anxiety disorder. A score of 10 or greater indicates threshold levels of anxiety that can be used for screening purposes. Cut points of 5, 10, and 15 are interpreted as a gradient of mild, moderate, and severe anxiety.

- **Patient-Reported Outcomes Measurement Information System (PROMIS®)**

  These measures evaluate self-reported symptoms including anxiety, depression, fatigue, sleep, and others. They are derived from legacy measures and have demonstrated validity in multiple settings including patients with cancer. PROMIS-anxiety comes as a short form, full length, or as computer adapted versions. Aside from background testing, another advantage to PROMIS is cross comparability to other symptom measures.

- **Death and Dying Distress Scale (DADDS)**

  A brief two-factor measure developed using patients with a prognosis greater than six months assessing:

  1. "Finitude of life"—fears about not having a future, running out of time, or being a burden;
  2. "Death-related distress"—worries or fears about the process of dying, such as death happening when alone, with a lot of pain or suffering, or being drawn out.

Clinical Management

Addressing anxiety in patients with advanced cancer or approaching the end of life should be tailored to the underlying cause (when possible), ongoing medical comorbidity, and preferences of the patient and family, while reassessing for efficacy. In general, a score of 10 or higher on the GAD-7 warrants attention. Treatment approaches should consider the underlying illness and prognosis, history of anxiety and past treatments, present psychosocial conditions, medical frailty, and other comorbidities. Treatment paradigms may be multilayered combining supportive care, psychotherapy, complementary and alternative therapies, and the judicious use of psychopharmacology.

Pharmacological Management of Anxiety Disorders

Medications have an important role in controlling symptoms of anxiety and anxiety disorders and are generally reserved for patients with greater severity of anxiety or functional impairment, who may require quicker responses, and are able to tolerate the side effects (see Table 2.2).

Several classes of medications have anxiolytic properties (e.g., anticonvulsants, neuroleptics, anticholinergic, and sedative/hypnotic medications) but benzodiazepines and antidepressants are the psychopharmacologic mainstay of treatment for acute and chronic anxiety. Management should address the underlying cause of anxiety and should be administered in a stepwise manner to prevent overtreatment and side effects, which may precipitate more anxiety.

- Benzodiazepines have demonstrated efficacy and tend to ameliorate anxiety quickly, which is beneficial for as-needed use. Benzodiazepines have

Table 2.2 Psychopharmacology of Selected Agents to Treat Anxiety in Advanced Cancer/End of Life Care

Medication	Route	Dosage	Half-Life (Hours)	Comments
Benzodiazepines				
Lorazepam	Oral, IM, IV	0.5–2.0mg daily, bd, tds, or qid	10–20	Metabolized by conjugation. Approved for chemotherapy-induced nausea & vomiting
Clonazepam	Oral	0.25–1.0 mg qhs, bd or tid	18–50	Seizure indications, relatively long acting
Diazepam	Oral, IV	2–10 mg bid–qid	30–100 (metabolites)	Anticonvulsant and muscle relaxant
Neuroleptic medications				
Olanzapine	Oral, or wafer	2.5–10 mg	21–54	Chemotherapy induced nausea; insomnia; weight gain
Quetiapine	Oral, IM	25–300 mg	7–12 (metabolite)	Sedation, augmentation for partial response to antidepressant or as monotherapy, rare tardive dyskinesia; antipsychotic choice in Parkinson's disease
Chlorpromazine	Oral, IM/IV	12.5–50 mg	30	Heavily sedating; QTc prolongation; useful for hiccups; hypotension; extrapyramidal side effects
First-line antidepressants—serotonin reuptake inhibitors				
Escitalopram	Oral	5–20 mg daily	25–30 hours	Mostly GI side effects, safe with tamoxifen
Citalopram	Oral	10–30 mg daily	35 hours	Safe in patients with seizures
Sertraline	Oral	50–200 mg daily	26 hours	Mostly GI side effects
Second-line antidepressants				
Mirtazapine	Oral	7.5–60mg qHS	20–40	Anxiety with insomnia, sedating, notably increases appetite
Buproprion	Oral	75–450 mg daily	7–12 (metabolite)	Smoking cessation, cancer related fatigue

Table 2.2 Continued

Medication	Route	Dosage	Half-Life (Hours)	Comments
Co-analgesic serotonin norepinephrine reuptake inhibitors				
Venlafaxine	Oral	37.5–300 mg daily	9–21 hours	Withdrawal syndrome, effective for hot flashes, safe with tamoxifen
Duloxetine	Oral	30–120 mg daily	12 hours	Useful for treatment of comorbid painful conditions; withdrawal if not tapered; risk of insomnia
Desvenlafaxine	Oral	25–150 mg daily	11 hours	Neuropathic pain
Anticonvulsant				
Pregabalin	Oral	50–300 mg	6.3	Onset within days; A GABA analog calcium channel modulator anticonvulsant; tolerance, dependence, and withdrawal are possible

Abbreviations: bid, twice per day; GABA, gamma-aminobutyric acid; IM, intramuscular; IV, intravenous; qHS, nightly; bd, twice a day; tid, three times a day; qid, four times a day

variable half-lives and excretion patterns that should be considered to prevent rebound anxiety and in patients with any evidence of or potential for organ failure.

• *Lorazepam* is generally favored in the hospital because it can be given orally or intravenously, has an 8- to 12-hour half-life, is not metabolized in the liver, and is consequently involved with less drug-–drug interactions (DDIs) than other benzodiazepines, which is clearly important for patients who are acutely ill.

  • *Midazolam* is used in syringe drivers in palliative care as its short half-life (2 hours) permits proportionate dose adjustment and it has proven compatibility with opioids delivered parenterally.

  • *Clonazepam* is used in tablet or liquid drop formulation in palliative care when a longer half-life of 24 + hours is desired to prevent rebound anxiety and a more potent formulation is needed in the benzodiazepine-tolerant patient.

Benzodiazepines are far safer in overdose than barbiturates and cause less respiratory suppression. But their effects are augmented by DDI and the presence of other psychoactive agents such as narcotics or alcohol. They need to be managed carefully with polypharmacy, and addiction potential should be thoroughly explained and reviewed.

🔍 Key Point

Antidepressant medications should be considered for patients with recurrent or chronic anxiety symptoms or disorders irrespective of the presence of depression. Antidepressants are anxiolytic but response onset may not begin for a few weeks and may require significant dose titration to achieve effect.

The choice of antidepressant depends most strongly on their side effect profiles. The selective serotonin reuptake inhibitors (SSRIs) are the class of choice given their efficacy and favorable side-effect profile in comparison to older antidepressant drug classes such as tricyclic antidepressants or mono-amine oxidase inhibitors (MAOIs). The SSRIs are much safer in the unfortunate event of an overdose and do not have the same anticholinergic or histaminic effects as the older classes of antidepressants. These side-effect profiles are especially important for patients with cancer who tend to be at risk of polypharmacy, side effects, and DDIs. The SSRIs can cause prolongation of the corrected QT interval (QTc) on the electrocardiogram (ECG), which may be especially important for hospitalized patients or those with electrolyte disturbances. As a class, they can cause hyponatremia and carry a mild risk of bleeding, along with dyspepsia. SSRIs can cause an activating effect that feels like restlessness (akathisia) but are often given concomitantly with an as-needed benzodiazepine, which may offset this effect.

Paroxetine is often chosen for patients with anxiety due to its sedating effect, but it carries more DDIs than other SSRIs, has anticholinergic properties, and may cause withdrawal symptoms with discontinuation. Escitalopram, citalopram, and sertraline may have the fewest DDIs, but they still need some consideration before prescribing them. Citalopram and escitalopram have greater risk for QTc prolongation and sertraline can cause or worsen gastrointestinal symptoms such as nausea and diarrhea. Fluoxetine has the longest half-life and therefore side effects will take longer to abate.

The serotonin-norepinephrine reuptake inhibitors (SNRIs) venlafaxine, desvenlafaxine, and duloxetine are indicated for anxiety and the treatment of neuropathic pain. Bupropion, an atypical antidepressant, is also indicated for anxiety and may be useful in ameliorating fatigue and asthenia. Mirtazapine, a tetracyclic antidepressant that antagonizes alpha 2 adrenergic receptors, has anxiolytic and sedative properties and the added benefit of appetite stimulation.

Other types of medications are often used in the management of anxiety in individuals with cancer and serious medical illnesses, even though they are not approved for this usage by regulatory agencies. These include medications used for pain or insomnia, like gabapentin, pregabalin, and trazodone (also an SSRI) because they have anxiolytic properties. Additionally, low-dose neuroleptic medications are sometimes prescribed when there is a contraindication for benzodiazepines (i.e., prior paradoxical reaction or concerns for worsening substance use) or anxiety refractory to benzodiazepines. Commonly used neuroleptics in this context include olanzapine, quetiapine, levomepromazine, and chlorpromazine. Patients with anxiety accompanied by agitation, delirium, psychosis, cognitive impairment ("sundowning") may benefit most immediately from administration of neuroleptic medications that antagonize dopamine receptors. These medications are particularly effective for patients at the end of life who are experiencing delirium.

Case Study 1

AB is a 59-year-old woman with a progressive adenocarcinoma of the lung who underwent a lobectomy 2 years prior to presentation. Approximately one year ago, she experienced lung cancer recurrence in both lungs and liver. She has been receiving a combination of immunotherapy and chemotherapy but appears to have advancing disease. In addition to a previous lung cancer surgery, her lungs show evidence of emphysema. She was a smoker for 30 years prior to her diagnosis. She has been hospitalized several times for pneumonia and other pulmonary symptoms. She reports increasing anxiety symptoms and panic attacks that may come out of nowhere but are also precipitated by exertion, certain body positions, or from coughing spells. She was recently prescribed home oxygen but finds it difficult to keep the nasal cannula on as she begins to feel claustrophobic. She has no history of anxiety or depression or other psychiatric disorders. She used to only feel anxious with dyspnea but now feels anxious all the time, she reflects on her diagnosis, worries about her family, having more symptoms, and has poor sleep. Her concentration is poor; she finds it difficult to engage with her treatment team. She fears becoming more anxious or having a panic attack. She denies depression or anhedonia.

In Case Study 1 (above), a small dose of opiate to alleviate breathlessness in a patient with advanced lung cancer and underlying lung disease may address the underlying or precipitating cause of her anxiety and lessen the need for anxiolytic medications. For this case, the approach should be stepwise with quick reassessments and consideration for starting and titrating a benzodiazepine for immediate management, starting an antidepressant for longer-term management of panic attacks, or even trying an alternate agent such as gabapentin if she has trouble tolerating a benzodiazepine. The patient reported panic attacks, so low-dose lorazepam could be used cautiously given her high risk of organ disfunction (i.e., respiratory suppression), DDI, and that a short-acting benzodiazepine such as alprazolam may cause rebound anxiety.

Psychological Therapies

Several psychological frameworks and related therapies have been applied to palliative care and end of life settings for the treatment of anxiety. For the most part, they can be grouped into psychoeducational, supportive, cognitive-behavioral therapy (CBT), and mind-body, existential, family-centered, or complementary treatment approaches. Each of these therapy approaches can be used for individuals, couples, families, and groups (see Chapter 7). The choice of psychological therapy should take into consideration the underlying cause of anxiety and precipitating factors. Previous therapies and their effectiveness should also be considered. Psychological therapies for anxiety tend to be focused on specific symptom control and gaining new coping tools or perspectives to alleviate anxiety.

Psychological interventions ought to be matched to the specific needs of patients rather than assuming that one or two methods can provide adequate efficacy across a broad range of needs. At the same time, the use of eHealth methods and training of palliative care nurses and other frontline allied healthcare professionals (AHPs) about anxiety interventions shows clinical benefits. Examples include lifestyle modifications (e.g., reducing caffeine intake, enhancing sleep hygiene protocols, obtaining regular exercise even when bedbound) and complementary therapies such as relaxation training, mindfulness meditation, and aromatherapy. Other complementary therapies may be available in palliative care services such as acupuncture, music or art therapy, and massage.

Overview of Psychological Interventions

This brief overview will focus on selected modalities that have demonstrated efficacy and are applicable to most clinical settings where patients with advanced cancer are treated.

Psychoeducational

These types of interventions vary in intensity of information. They range from intensive training in coping skills, health education, and supportive techniques to briefer forms of psychoeducation as part of an information orientation. Skills-based approaches are more efficacious than information-only programs.[12] These skill-based, psychoeducational approaches reduce anxiety by helping patients master new knowledge about their cancer and effectively alleviates aspects of uncertainty. The unknown elements of cancer and its treatments challenge the coping abilities of all patients. Psychoeducational interventions may be combined with other therapies.

🔍 Key Points

Some of the key educational components are highlighted below:

- Review of emotional reaction to the prognosis
- Normalizing grief, empathizing with it, yet considering its burdensomeness in the time that remains
- Coming to terms with uncertainty and helping to accept cancer and its implications
- Teasing out the focus of fears (what's behind the fear)
- Active discussion of the likely mode of dying (e.g., death by liver failure) and how palliative treatments ensure a peaceful dying process
- Being educative about symptom management options for pain, breathlessness, insomnia, and other common symptoms at the end of life
- Realignment of hope into a "here and now" focus
- Identification of tasks that remain, concerns that can be addressed, goodbyes that can be shared

- Identification of relationships that matter, family needs, unfinished business
- Introduction of chaplains or pastoral care workers to alleviate religious concerns.

Psychoeducational interventions are applied to all cancer types and treatment settings. These interventions can be delivered in-person, via video, or print media and by a clinical treatment team, nurse, administrator, or physician.

Time-Limited Cognitive-Behavioral Therapy (CBT)

CBT can be used to treat anxiety with various patient types and settings. CBT has been studied extensively, but the approach presents some challenges as it is translated for cancer settings. For patients with cancer, the approach should be tailored or adapted to the realities and expectations of the cancer situation. Traditionally, CBT focuses on thought processes e.g., negative automatic thoughts (NATs) and behaviors that can be identified and reframed in a more adaptive way. Thoughts are no longer evaluated for their logic or rationality but rather for how helpful or constructive they are for the clinical circumstances. Care must be taken to understand the clinical context so that the clinician does not invalidate realistic worries about actual losses, functional impairment, or even death. An approach to understanding the thought processes and distinctions between real and exaggerated responses is therapeutic while also focusing on enhancing acceptance and toleration of distress as clinically appropriate.

Behaviorally oriented elements of CBT may be particularly beneficial for patients with advanced cancer and include; short-term, goal-focused problem-solving, relaxation techniques, and CBT for specific problems such as insomnia (CBTi). Within the CBT framework, goal-setting needs to provide a short-term focus so patients can achieve a sense of progress and relief of anxiety within a realistic timeframe.

Other behavioral approaches for specific phobias or traumas include guided exposure and systematic desensitization. These can be particularly useful modalities to lessen anxiety provided there is a realistic timeframe for implementation. Many systematic desensitization programs need a period of adaptive learning that limits their use in those receiving end of life care. It is also important to first assess patient motivation and physical capacity in those patients with advanced cancer.

🔍 Key Points
- Behavioral and cognitive components of CBT effectively address psychological symptoms such as anxiety that are highly prevalent at the end of life.
- Relaxation techniques, guided imagery, breathing exercises may alleviate anxiety symptoms
- NATs may be assessed not primarily for their irrationality but for how helpful or unhelpful they are.

Mindfulness-Based Stress Reduction (MBSR)

Examine prior use of relaxation and mindfulness techniques to assess for likely gains from upskilling in the palliative care setting. A present-oriented focus and attention is used in mindfulness to create a heightened sense of awareness and deliberate attention to physical and mental state. This practice emphasizes nonjudging awareness and acceptance and has been shown to mitigate anxiety symptoms in patients with cancer.[13] Eight-week training sessions are available for patients to learn MBSR techniques and can be done in-person or online. These trainings are experiential as well as psychoeducational, providing trainees with experiential learning that is meant to be incorporated into one's lifestyle.

Dignity Therapy (DT)

DT is an individualized and brief psychotherapy that can be done in one or more sessions. Many palliative care services use volunteers trained as biographers to do this. Patients are given a set of nine questions to reflect on prior to sessions, which are recorded and transcribed into a legacy document. DT aims to relieve existential distress and improve the experiences of those whose lives are threatened by cancer.[14] It can be adapted for patients with physical limitations.

Meaning-Centered Therapy (MCP)

MCP is a brief multisession individual or group psychotherapy that targets existential distress and despair.[15] It is based on the fundamental elements of Victor Frankl's logotherapy as described in his seminal book, *Man's Search for Meaning*. MCP requires intensive training and has been adapted to myriad palliative settings in many languages.

Managing Cancer and Living Meaningfully (CALM)

CALM is a three- to eight-session intervention grounded in "relational, attachment and existential theory" that can be delivered in-person, by telephone, or by a virtual platform. It is semistructured and focuses on four key domains: symptom control and communication with healthcare providers; self-concept and relations with others; spiritual well-being and the values and beliefs that provide meaning and purpose in life; and preparing for the future, sustaining hope, and facing mortality. It has demonstrated efficacy in ameliorating death anxiety, depression, and other psychological symptoms and increasing spiritual well-being in patients with advanced cancer.[16]

Family-Centered Therapy Techniques

Family meetings can be employed regularly to ameliorate anxiety in family members using psychoeducational and supportive techniques. Caregiver fear and anxiety negatively affects patients and caregivers alike, especially as relationships are strained by end of life stressors. Palliative care services may provide these services in collaboration with mental health services.

Case Study 2

An 82-year-old man with advanced prostate cancer has just started on hospice care. He is experiencing anxiety about not receiving specific anticancer treatment and is having initial insomnia, early wakefulness, and waking up in a cold sweat. He is not able to relax. Although he does not want any more side effects from anticancer treatments, he is nervous about the limited amount of time he has left to live. He wants to enjoy this time with his family. But persistent anxiety does not allow him to have the peace that he would like to have. He feels his mood continues to deteriorate, which brings frustration. He denies depression and does not have any history of mood or psychotic disorders. He has only just started an increased dose of narcotic-based pain medication and is reluctant to take medications for his anxiety, since he feels it could cloud his senses. Interview sessions reveal that he is worried that he has not accomplished all that he set out to do and wants to provide more financial security for his wife and children.

The Case 2 patient may be helped by a brief psychotherapeutic modality that functions as a life review and is adaptive for meaningful living in the present moment. Dignity therapy, MCP, or CALM would be good choices. A focused session on his role within his family using the principles of dignity therapy may provide a new therapeutic perspective. If he expressed existential despair and regret, MCP may be the most appropriate choice. CALM could also be used to understand his self-concept at this stage of his life in relation to his family and other people who are important to him. Case 2 may benefit from addressing past accomplishments and their meanings as well as planning on what can be done in the moment and alleviating any hidden sources of anxiety.

Professional Issues and Service Implementation

Multidisciplinary Teams

Working within multidisciplinary cancer treatment teams should be a priority to meet the needs of comprehensive care of patients at the end of life. For this reason, mental health professionals should be included as part of the wider medical management team in any oncology care facility. This will enable the provision of gold standard comprehensive cancer care, especially within the context of palliative care or end of life care.

Recording and Communicating

The following points should be helpful:

- Ideally there should be agreed procedures, in law, for recording discussions of advanced directives or requests for assisted dying (see Chapters 1 and 6).
- Access by family members to confidential information, provided by patients, needs to follow an agreed national, legal, or organizational policy.
- Communication with family caregivers and relatives should be recorded, especially if there are anxiety issues that may affect the patient, end of life care, and the treatment team.
- The role of anxiety, in impacting decision-making by patients, needs to be recorded where appropriate.
- All treatments for anxiety should be recorded in the appropriate medical notes.

- Communication of details of anxiety and any treatments, to other professionals, needs to follow duty of care requirements and should be in the patient's best interests.

Where patients want to record their therapy sessions with their providers, this should be discussed and examined prior to beginning a therapy session. Patient and therapists should agree on recording or not recording, and attempts should be made to find out what this method of communication means for the patient. Effort should be made to communicate clearly with patients and offer alternate modes of communication that might be more comfortable or appropriate.

The therapist should have a clear idea of their interpersonal boundaries to guide these discussions. For example, email is a comfortable for some therapists but not all therapists. It can raise important issues outside of the context of therapy. Also, therapist involvement on social media should be limited to what might be acceptable for a patient to witness. Therapists need to make decisions about patients who desire contact in these arenas. "Friend requests" and other socially inclusive methods of communication need to be openly discussed and agreed upon within the therapy session. Therapists should also discuss these modes of communication in their own supervision to proactively manage any possible nontherapeutic disclosures and other issues.

Legal Responsibilities

Where there is a need for patient restraint, for the purpose of managing anxiety or agitation, local/national laws should be followed to avoid harm to frail patients. Attention from a one-on-one nursing specialist may be more helpful than physical restraints.

Confidentiality

Managing patients with advanced cancer who may be encountering end of life issues requires exceptional respect for privacy and confidentiality. This is the bedrock of the therapeutic setting and demonstrates respect for the patient and their family.

Known Mental Illness

Patients with known serious mental illness have a distinct set of needs in the palliative care or end of life setting. The management of primary psychiatric disorders should be concurrent. It may be necessary to pay extra attention to informed decision-making to ensure that the patient's wishes and values are represented and respected. Assessment of competency, where there is known serious mental illness, may need to be established within national legal requirements. Communication is crucial among the various healthcare professionals involved in the patient's care. Psychiatric decompensation can derail successful palliation of symptoms and cancer care.

Cultural Issues

An understanding of cultural/religious/spiritual issues as they affect levels of anxiety is important as these beliefs need to be considered and integrated into care (see Chapter 9). There is no cookbook list for management except to say that training in awareness of these issues, especially in multicultural and multiethnic contexts, usually improves end of life and palliative care experiences for patients and their families/caregivers. Issues that impact the patient's experience of anxiety can be linked to spiritual and cultural beliefs about death and dying. In some instances, families may be helpful when it comes to interpreting either high levels of anxiety or a lack of appropriate worry linked to these beliefs. Online training can improve skills and facilitate appropriate clinical decisions. Useful websites that provide management guidance are listed at the end of the chapter.

Policies and Protocols

All centers where palliative or end of life care is provided will need a policy on the management of clinical anxiety for their patients. A flowchart is helpful in guiding staff on the protocols and decision-making required.

Teams and Supervision

Ideally, teams should follow a multidisciplinary model that includes and provides input, not only from the direct palliative medical and nursing team but also the following professionals: psychiatrists, clinical psychologists, counseling psychologists, chaplaincy, social services, and bereavement specialists.

Where possible, regular supervision, according to local practices, should integrate discussion of psychosocial dimensions of patients care with specific attention to clinical anxiety and depression as well as any safety issues.

The effects of patient and caregiver anxiety on clinicians and their countertransference reactions should be anticipated and considered among treatment teams.

References

1. Mitchell AJ, Chan M, Bhatti H, et al. Prevalence of depression, anxiety, and adjustment disorder in oncological, haematological, and palliative-care settings: A meta-analysis of 94 interview-based studies. Lancet Oncol. 2011;12(2): 160–174. https://doi.org/10.1016/S1470-2045(11)70002-X.

2. Oechsle K, Ullrich A, Marx G, et al. Psychological burden in family caregivers of patients with advanced cancer at initiation of specialist inpatient palliative care. BMC Palliat Care. 2019;18(1):102. https://doi.org/10.1186/s12904-019-0469-7.

3. Selamat Din SH, Nik Jaafar NR., Zakaria H, Mohamed Saini S, Ahmad SN, Midin M. Anxiety disorders in family caregivers of breast cancer patients receiving oncologic treatment in Malaysia. Asian Pac J Cancer Prev. 2017;18(2):465–471. https://doi.org/10.22034/APJCP.2017.18.2.465.

4. Linden W, Vodermaier A, Mackenzie R, Greig D. Anxiety and depression after cancer diagnosis: Prevalence rates by cancer type, gender, and age. J Affect Disord. 2012;141(2–3):343–351. https://doi.org/10.1016/j.jad.2012.03.025.

5. Neel C, Lo C, Rydall A, Hales S, Rodin G. Determinants of death anxiety in patients with advanced cancer. BMJ Support Palliat Care. 2015;5(4):373–380. https://doi.org/10.1136/bmjspcare-2012-000420.

6. Costello H, Gould RL, Abrol E, Howard R. Systematic review and meta-analysis of the association between peripheral inflammatory cytokines and generalised anxiety disorder. BMJ Open. 2019;9(7):e027925. https://doi.org/10.1136/bmjopen-2018-027925.

7. Haroon E, Miller AH, Sanacora, G. Inflammation, glutamate, and glia: A trio of trouble in mood disorders. Neuropsychopharmacology. 2017;42(1):193–215. https://doi.org/10.1038/npp.2016.199.

8. Mitchell AJ, Rao S, Vaze A. Can general practitioners identify people with distress and mild depression? A meta-analysis of clinical accuracy. J Affect Disord. 2011;130(1–2):26–36. https://doi.org/10.1016/j.jad.2010.07.028.

9. McFarland DC, Jutagir DR, Miller A, Nelson, C. Physical problem list accompanying the distress thermometer: Its associations with psychological symptoms and survival in patients with metastatic lung cancer. Psycho-Oncology. 2020;29(5):910–919. https://doi.org/10.1002/pon.5367.

10. Lawlor PG, Gagnon B, Mancini IL, et al. Occurrence, causes, and outcome of delirium in patients with advanced cancer: A prospective study. Arch Intern Med. 2000;160(6):786–794. https://doi.org/10.1001/archinte.160.6.786.

11. Ahn MH, Park S, Lee HB, et al. Suicide in cancer patients within the first year of diagnosis. Psycho-Oncology. 2015;24(5):601–607. https://doi.org/10.1002/pon.3705.

12. Faller H, Schuler M, Richard M, Heckl U, Weis J, Kuffner R. Effects of psychooncologic interventions on emotional distress and quality of life in adult patients with cancer: Systematic review and meta-analysis. J Clin Oncol. 2013;31(6):782–793. https://doi.org/10.1200/JCO.2011.40.8922.

13. Cillessen L, Johannsen M, Speckens AEM, Zachariae R. Mindfulness-based interventions for psychological and physical health outcomes in cancer patients and survivors: A systematic review and meta-analysis of randomized controlled trials. Psychooncology. 2019;28(12):2257–2269. https://doi.org/10.1002/pon.5214.

14. Martinez M, Arantzamendi M, Belar, A, et al. "Dignity therapy" a promising intervention in palliative care: A comprehensive systematic literature review. Palliat Med. 2017;31(6):492–509. https://doi.org/10.1177/0269216316665562.

15. Breitbart W, Pessin H, Rosenfeld B, et al. Individual meaning-centered psychotherapy for the treatment of psychological and existential distress: A randomized controlled trial in patients with advanced cancer. Cancer. 2018;124(15):3231–3239. https://doi.org/10.1002/cncr.31539.

16. Lo C, Hales S, Jung J, et al. Managing Cancer And Living Meaningfully (CALM): Phase 2 trial of a brief individual psychotherapy for patients with advanced cancer. Palliat Med. 2014;28(3):234–242. https://doi.org/10.1177/0269216313507757.

Further Reading

Cherny NI, Fallon MT, Kaasa S, Portenoy RK, Currow DC, Editors. Oxford Textbook of Palliative Medicine. 6th ed. Oxford: Oxford University Press; 2021. This has an excellent chapter on anxiety disorders in the palliative and end of life setting.

Nelson AM, Rapaport CS, Traeger L, Greer JA. Anxiety disorders. In Psycho-Oncology. 4th ed. W. S. Breitbart et al., Editors. New York: Oxford University Press; 2020. Pages 338–344. This is recommended as a brief chapter on anxiety disorders across the disease spectrum.

Roth AJ. Anxiety in palliative care. In Handbook of Psychiatry in Palliative Medicine. 3rd ed. Harvey Max Chochinov and William S. Breitbart, Editors. Oxford: Oxford University Press, 2022. This is recommended as a chapter on anxiety that is focused on the palliative care setting.

Useful Websites
- American Cancer Society-Emotional, Mental Health and Mood Changes

https://www.cancer.org/treatment/treatments-and-side-effects/physical-side-effects/emotional-mood-changes/anxiety.html

- End of life ESSENTIALS—educational modules for clinicians

https://www.endoflifeessentials.com.au/tabid/5195/Default.aspx

- National Comprehensive Cancer Network Distress Guidelines

https://www.nccn.org/guidelines/guidelines-detail?category=3&id=1431

- National Comprehensive Cancer Network Distress for Patients

https://www.nccn.org/patients/guidelines/content/PDF/distress-patient.pdf

Chapter 3

Adjustment Disorder and Demoralization

David W. Kissane, Luigi Grassi, and Chun-Kai Fang

Learning Objectives

After reading this chapter, the clinician will be able to:

1. Describe the prevalence and diagnostic criteria for the states of adjustment disorder and demoralization in palliative care;
2. Identify risk factors for their development alongside protective factors that sustain resilience and adaptive coping, and the place of assessment and screening methods to enhance recognition;
3. List strategies to ameliorate demoralization, enhance adjustment and treat patients who develop clinical disorders, including suicidal thinking;
4. Describe ethical, cultural, legal and professional issues which may arise in the clinical care of patients with adjustment disorder or demoralization.

Background Evidence

The Traditional View of Adjustment Disorder

Adjustment disorder (AD) refers to a diagnosis recognized in the psychiatric nosological systems as a stress-response syndrome, namely a maladaptive reaction to an identifiable stressor. As such, it identifies poor coping. AD has appeared in psychiatric classification systems for over 50 years under varied names like "situational crisis," and since DSM-III and ICD-10, the language of "adjustment disorder" was settled on.[1]

The necessary ICD-11 and DSM-5-TR criteria for a diagnosis of Adjustment Disorder can be summarized as:

- The distress should be intense, preoccupying, and out of proportion to what would be expected, with excessive worry or rumination about what will happen;
- The resultant poor coping causes functional impairment in living, work, social relationships, or other key aspects of functioning; and
- The onset follows a stressful event, diagnosis, or disease progression, typically within 3 months and the disorder improves by 6 months.

For ICD-11, Adjustment Disorder (code 6B43) has many possible synonyms, including brief situational nonpsychotic disorder, adaptation reaction not otherwise specified, adjustment reaction, emotional crisis, situational disorder or maladjustment or situational reaction with maladjustment, transient situational disturbance, and embitterment reaction. It is excluded by other diagnoses, including single episode or recurrent depressive disorder, uncomplicated bereavement, prolonged grief disorder, and burnout. Recent indications from the Global Clinical Practice Network (GCP) suggest that symptoms of preoccupation tend to worsen with any reminder of the stressor/diagnosis, resulting in avoidant coping—avoidance of stimuli, thoughts, feelings, or discussions associated with the stressor to prevent further preoccupation or suffering. Also, additional psychological symptoms include a range of depressive or anxiety symptoms, as well as impulsive "externalizing" symptoms, such as increased tobacco, alcohol, or other substance use. Finally, individuals with AD usually recover when the stressor is removed, when sufficient support is provided, or when the person develops more adaptive coping mechanisms or strategies.

For DSM-5-TR, with Adjustment Disorder (code 309.9), specifiers are used to delineate subtypes that may guide better recognition and treatment choice—AD with depressed mood, with anxiety, with mixed anxiety and depressed mood, with disturbance of conduct, with mixed disturbance of emotions and conduct, and not otherwise specified (NOS).[2] Symptoms can result from a single event or continually stressful circumstances. ADs are associated with increased suicidality. In contrast with DSM-5, ICD-11 has removed the use of specifiers for AD, preferring a unifaceted concept of adjustment disorder that varies only by symptom severity.

The Concept of Demoralization

Demoralization is a state of poor coping characterized by symptoms of low morale, hopelessness, sense of entrapment, and loss of meaning and purpose in life. As such, the concept matches the criteria for AD, yet it brings key phenomena of existential distress to enrich any diagnostic criteria in the palliative care setting. There is a long literature describing this construct, including classic writings by George Engel, Viktor Frankl, and Jerome Frank. It is common in palliative care, with its recognition building in parallel with Susan Folkman recognizing the importance of meaning-based coping, alongside emotion-based and problem-based responses to stressful illnesses such as AIDS. The development of a validated measure and its translation into 20 languages saw its recognition as a clinical syndrome that can be differentiated from depression.[3] While demoralization has been well studied in oncology and palliative care settings, it is also common in other medical and mental illnesses, refugees, substance users, adolescents, the postnatal period and in adjustment to stressors like relationship breakdown.

Prevalence of Adjustment Disorder and Demoralization

Studies in the medically ill have shown a 15% prevalence of AD, with a further 10% identified as possible cases both in the United States and Europe. In cancer patients, by using different versions of the DSM and the ICD, ADs were found in 15% to 20% depending on phases of illness.[4]

The prevalence of demoralization identified in systematic reviews includes 15% of palliative care patients,[5] 25% of medically ill patients,[6] and up to 50% of psychiatrically ill patients.[6] Such prevalences have not only highlighted its importance, but these reviews have also clarified its differentiation from depression.[7]

Critique of Adjustment Disorder

Much criticism has been raised about the diagnosis of AD, such as a lack of validation of or ambiguity in its symptom structure, the nonspecificity and instability of symptoms, and the timeframe (6 months or, in exceptional cases, 2 years after termination of the stressor), which is generally not helpful for chronic stress conditions. Also, some have criticized the distance from the real clinical world of the six "specific" subtypes[8] of AD (as in DSM-5) or little support for the two-symptom structure used in ICD-11.[9] Others consider that the diagnostic category should be retained because it serves a useful clinical purpose for clinicians seeking a temporary, mild, nonstigmatizing diagnosis for health insurance purposes.[10]

The problem of making a diagnosis of AD in medical settings is part of this debate, since psychiatric nosological systems fail to provide clear-enough diagnostic criteria that guide clinicians in distinguishing AD from normal adaptive reactions to physical disease (particularly chronic somatic illnesses, which are the majority), on the one hand, or from subthreshold mental disorders (e.g., depression, other subsyndromal stress disorders), on the other.

AD diagnostic criteria are not easy to apply to a chronic situation such as cancer. In one study of 800 medically ill patients, including cancer patients, those who received a diagnosis of adjustment disorder (12%) were characterized by many different dimensions, including health anxiety, demoralization, alexithymia, illness denial, persistent somatization, and irritable mood, which are only partially or not at all overlapping with the DSM subtypes.[11] At the same time, those affected by major depression (12.7%) could be classified as depressed somatizers or irritable/anxious depression.

Demoralization as a Form of Adjustment Disorder

The importance of recognizing demoralization clinically lies in the specificity of its symptoms in capturing maladaptive coping, the therapeutic target these symptoms become in treatment approaches, its strong association with suicidal thinking (independently of anhedonia), and its prominent prevalence, well illustrated in this setting of palliative care. When a latent class analysis was applied to a cohort of 1,527 patients with cancer, moderate demoralization clustered with symptoms of adjustment disorder.[12] When a network approach to psychopathology was applied to a medically ill cohort, symptoms of anhedonic depression clearly separated from symptoms of demoralization, with suicidal thoughts belonging strongly to the demoralization community of symptoms.[13] Such studies support the differentiation of demoralization (coping) from depression (anhedonia).

Risk Factors for Demoralization

Risk factors for demoralization include:
- physical and mental illnesses with high symptom burdens that challenge coping
- burdensome treatments

- prolonged or repeated hospitalizations
- poorer education and health literacy
- lower income and socioeconomic deprivation
- being female
- single status (unmarried, separated, divorced, widowed)
- lacking social supports.

The enduring human need for dignity and meaning in life transcends cultures and highlights the salience of sense-making and relationships to human well-being. Demoralization is therefore integrated into this chapter on AD in an effort to enrich our understanding of its symptom profile and treatment, given its strong association with AD.

Evidence for the Treatment of Adjustment Disorder and Demoralization in Palliative Care

Surprisingly, a formal evidence base for the management of AD in palliative care patients is absent, both because of the more dominant focus on anxiety and mood disorders, and the challenge in accurately diagnosing AD. Clinical consensus would advocate for the use of supportive, cognitively oriented and meaning-centered psychotherapies, and the latter have proved helpful when existential distress is present.[14] Thus, the randomized trial of individual meaning-centered psychotherapy (IMCP) showed small to medium effects in improving sense of meaning and spiritual well-being.

The Managing Cancer and Living Meaningfully (CALM) therapy trial[15] had depressive symptoms as its primary outcome, but among secondary outcomes, when death anxiety was high at baseline (i.e., existential distress was present), CALM showed a moderate effect size in improving demoralization, spiritual well-being, and relieving death anxiety. More recent trials of psilocybin-assisted psychotherapy, which aim to enhance meaning, have also revealed benefits in reducing demoralization.[16,17]

Taken together, this evidence base offers great promise for the role of meaning-centered therapies in ameliorating demoralization, and by extension, helping to assuage AD.

Presenting Problems

Patients may not always recognize that their illness, its treatment, disease progression, the prognosis, or symptoms that prove troublesome, can be seen as a stressor that is a challenge to their coping. Nevertheless, this is often the case. The medical predicament challenges their coping, causing grief and potentially lowering their morale.

Key Symptoms and Signs

The common symptoms of AD and demoralization include:

- Distress, upset, grief, and sadness
- Low morale, feeling disheartened, discouraged, losing confidence about treatment

- Sense of poor coping, feeling a failure, struggling to cope with the illness
- Feeling trapped by the illness, stuck, with growing helplessness
- Hopelessness, pessimistic about the future
- Pointlessness and meaninglessness, loss of the value of life
- Purposelessness, loss of direction, loss of goals
- Feeling alone, isolated, or alienated from others
- Loss of roles, creativity, ways of gaining fulfillment, including relationships
- Loss of self-worth, loss of dignity, embarrassment or shame
- Loss of control, not feeling choices are yours to make
- Other dysphoric emotions including irritability and anger
- Resultant impairment in functioning, social withdrawal
- Ruminating about all of this and despairing
- Readiness to give up on life, desire death, or wish to hasten death
- Suicidal plans

Alongside these symptoms, key signs include:

- Waves of tearfulness, yet ability to rally again
- Reactivity of affects is retained, smiling freely
- Sense of humor persists, with spontaneous laughter evident
- Ability to enjoy visitors, reading or follow entertainment
- Interest in activities and enjoyment of pleasurable things
- Cognitive function is intact, fully oriented, memory reasonable, judgment sound
- Health literacy may not be great, with limited understanding of prognosis
- Insight into loss of morale and hope is generally present

AD, with maladaptive coping, can be seen with a predominant affect such as anxious or depressed mood, or with behavioral disturbance. In the DSM system, these are designated "specifiers" because they enrich understanding and guide the choice of treatment. Thus, when depressive symptoms are present, the diagnosis in DSM-5 would be Adjustment Disorder with Depressed Mood. When the symptoms of demoralization predominate, with low morale, sense of poor coping, entrapment,

---

Box 3.1 Diagnostic Criteria for Adjustment Disorder (Blending ICD-11 and DSM-5-TR Criteria)

The formal diagnosis of an Adjustment Disorder is based on recognition of:

1. the illness as a stressor that challenges coping;
2. the presence of distressing symptoms out of proportion to what is expected from the predicament;
3. a timeline linking the symptoms to the stressor/illness; and
4. maladaptive coping resulting in impairment in personal, family, social, educational, occupational, or other important areas of functioning.

hopelessness, or pointlessness, the use of a specifier could be similarly employed, with a formal diagnosis being "Adjustment Disorder with Demoralization."

In the cancer and palliative care setting, clinicians can hesitate to offer the diagnosis of "Adjustment Disorder" as it can appear to be a hurtful label with a pejorative dimension. However, patients readily acknowledge low morale and feeling demoralized, such that the direct use of this construct, with words like "feeling demoralized," allows supportive counseling and treatment to be planned. In this sense, some clinicians prefer to offer a diagnosis of Demoralization Syndrome in preference to AD, while others simply use the word "Demoralization" to describe what they see happening in the patient. The word "demoralization" proves to be readily accepted and understood by patients, clinical teams, and families alike. Demoralization is well covered in textbooks of psycho-oncology and palliative medicine, but is still to be adopted by psychiatric classification systems. Where clinicians adopt this approach, the following Box 3.2 offers key diagnostic criteria.

Moreover, the phenomenology of demoralization described in the symptoms above achieves a much richer gestalt of the patient's experience than that found in the diagnostic lists for AD. Scholars have recognized the unidimensionality of symptoms associated with poor coping as seen in demoralization, its comorbidity with other mental illnesses, its vital importance in treatment planning, and its seriousness as a mediator of suicide.

Precipitating Factors
Typical issues that precipitate these symptoms and signs include:
- Exhaustion of anticancer treatments to contain or slow disease progression
- Poor symptom control—debilitating physical symptoms, which can be refractory to treatment and unrelenting in nature, e.g., pain, nausea, vomiting, breathlessness, fatigue, insomnia, itch, hiccup, and so on.
- Incontinence of urine and faeces

Box 3.2 Diagnostic Criteria for Demoralization

A formal diagnosis of Demoralization is based on the following key symptoms being present for two or more weeks:
1. Low morale, feeling disheartened or discouraged
2. Sense of poor coping, not managing, or feeling a failure
3. Feeling trapped, stuck, or unable to change the predicament
4. Hopeless, pessimistic about the future
5. Pointlessness, with loss of meaning, value, and purpose in life
6. Resultant excessive distress or impairment in functioning in normal roles
7. Potential for suicidal thoughts or plans

- Skin breakdown, with wounds, bedsore, smelly odor
- Falls with fractures, loss of mobility, loss of safety as an independent person
- Cachexia, weight loss, weakness, and fatigue
- Debility from deconditioning, rendering the patient chairbound, and then bedbound
- Stroke, paralysis, limb weakness, and loss of functionality
- Blindness or deafness, loss of other senses
- Cognitive decline with memory failure, dysphasia, attentional deficits, loss of executive or planning functions
- Hemorrhage, pancytopenia, incipient organ failure
- Awareness that death is drawing closer

Predisposing Factors

Typical predisposing issues that are located in the background, temperament, and character of the person include:

- Attachment insecurity
- Low self-esteem, self-doubt
- Neurotic traits, worrying all one's life
- Single status as separated, divorced, widowed, never married
- Relational difficulties, isolation and alienation, family breakdown
- Poverty and financial hardship, often a struggle to manage
- Social displacement, migrant, refugee status
- Chronic mental illness, chronic dysthymia, treatment-resistant depression
- Chronic disability, poor physical health, cumulative chronic illness
- Limited education and poor health literacy
- Language barriers
- Previous traumas
- Spiritual or religious angst and doubt

Perpetuating Factors

Typical problems that cause persistence or recurrence of the situation include:

- Dysfunctional family, carers not coping, feeling unsupported
- Dependent children, disabled children, unable to meet responsibilities to loved ones
- Relentless disease progression, with unstable or deteriorating symptom control
- Communication breakdown, not feeling understood
- Experience of physician abandonment, unavailability, doubt about expertise
- Unrecognized and untreated mental illness
- Unidentified existential or spiritual distress

Protective Factors

Strengths of the person are vital to identify and include:

- Resilient character strengths with strong education, maturity, wisdom
- Coherent narrative of a fulfilling and creative life
- Strong religious belief and availability of a faith community
- Supportive network of family and friends
- Open communication, openness to new experience, adaptability, and flexibility

Case Study

Jessica is a 50-year-old divorcee and single mother who has worked as a town planner. She developed a small bowel obstruction from extrinsic pressure arising from peritoneal nodules associated with a BRAF-mutated colorectal cancer. Her oncologist conveyed pessimism about her prospects of recovery, although treatment with cetuximab and encorafenib had just started. Jessica had struggled with nausea and vomiting over a couple of months, leaving her malnourished and in a stressful predicament. A palliative care physician asked if she wanted to forgo further immunotherapy as she seemed quite frail, but Jessica was motivated to see her daughter's Prom! She asked for total parenteral nutrition to sustain her for a time longer. After one month, her CEA tumor marker was lower and nodule size had decreased on imaging. Her physicians agreed to feed her parenterally.

Jessica was quite thin, yet managed a warm smile as she watched from her hospital bed. She acknowledged that she had felt quite discouraged in recalling her oncologist's concern that treatment might not help her quickly enough. The surgeon had considered her inoperable. No-one held much hope, leaving Jessica feeling trapped in a situation she could not control. Her daughter had pleaded with the team to continue treatment, and her mother's CEA levels continued to fall. Jessica commented that when the doctors seemed to have given up, it was hard to hold on to hope.

The nurse asked Jessica how she was feeling. Jessica denied feeling depressed. She kept her sense of humor and thrived on family visitors. She had felt rather weak and fatigued before the TPN started but was sleeping soundly enough. She volunteered that she hoped one day her bowel would wake up! For a while, she had wondered what the point was, and realized that her morale was very low, struggling to keep hope alive. But then the immune therapy seemed to be working.

Investigations for Key Differential Diagnoses

Differential Diagnoses to Consider

When the affective symptoms are being thought about, the clinician differentiates the variable pattern of emotions that come in waves and are fleeting from the pervasive pattern of depressed mood and anhedonia that persists across the day and for longer than two weeks in

- **Major Depressive Episode**, or variations like Major Depression with Melancholia, or Major Depression with Psychotic Features;

When unhappiness is chronic and long-lasting, often longer than two years, and the cluster of symptoms is fewer, a diagnosis is made of
• **Dysthymia**;
With these affective disorders, psychiatric classification systems have not paid strong attention to any associated deficits of coping that accompany the clinical depression, but this comorbidity is the norm and symptoms of demoralization are found to result from depressive disorders.

When symptoms of anxiety, worry, or rumination predominate, and when this follows a life-long pattern of worrying, the differential diagnosis is
• **Generalized Anxiety Disorder**;
When symptoms of anxiety occur as discrete episodes of panic, with associated features of palpitations, breathlessness, tremor and sweating, the differential diagnosis is
• **Panic Disorder**; or variations like Panic Disorder with Agoraphobia;
When symptoms of anxiety are directed to a specific object, such as a needle, then the differential diagnosis is
• **Phobia**, or variations such as Needle Phobia;

In association with these anxiety symptoms, psychiatric classification systems have not paid strong attention to any associated deficits of coping that accompany anxiety disorders, but this comorbidity is the norm and symptoms of demoralization are found to result from anxiety disorders.

When an event has been unexpectedly terrifying and traumatic, such that it induced dissociative symptoms over the next three or more days, including numbing, sense of unreality, and loss of recall of the event, and includes flashbacks, hyperarousal, startle responses, nightmares, and intense reactions to cues of the event, the differential diagnosis is
• **Acute Stress Disorder**, or with persistence of these symptoms beyond the month, Posttraumatic Stress Disorder;
The nature of such traumatic events is generally very different from an illness experience, and includes events like fires, earthquakes, assaults, or motor vehicle accidents that might constitute an immediate threat to life. The existential threat found in palliative care is more continual, may have developed insidiously with disease progression, and is uncommonly associated with the dissociation and hyperarousal found in these stress disorder responses.

Key Investigations to Consider

Some psychosocial clinicians may need to liaise with other appropriate disciplines for guidance about some of the investigations discussed in this section. All clinicians, however, need to consider biopsychosocial and spiritual contributions to the clinical picture and understand when to ask their colleagues for help. From the biomedical perspective, a number of medical factors can contribute to the symptoms of adjustment and demoralization as assessed in what follows:
• Electrolytes (Na+, K+, Mg++, Ca++), Urea, Creatinine for poor sense of well-being, fatigue
• Full Blood Examination for anaemia if fatigue is prominent

- Thyroid function (T4, TSH) when fatigue, tremor, and weight change are concerning
- Nutritional deficiencies (B1, B6, B12, Vit C, Folate, Fe) when cachexia and fatigue are prominent
- ECG, QTc interval, if medications (e.g., neuroleptics, SSRIs, opioids) may interact
- Imaging (Xray, CT, MRI, PET) when assessment of prognosis or pain physiology is required
- Functional assessment may be needed if safety and self-care capacity is required: Occupational and physical therapy assessments
- Spiritual well-being assessment is achieved by the referral to chaplaincy or pastoral care
- Family support and carer assessment may be required: Social worker or family clinic may be needed.

Severity Assessment for Treatment Planning and Follow-Up

Adjustment Disorder Structured Interview

Assessment of AD has always represented a problem because of the lack of studies regarding valid and reliable measures and the vagueness of the definition of the syndrome in DSM and ICD. Recently, in agreement with the reconceptualization and creation of ICD-11 criteria, a self-report Adjustment Disorder-New Module (ADNM) was developed and validated in an original 20-item form,[18,19] but also in shorter 8- (Brief) and 4-item (Ultra Brief) forms to be used as screening tools.[20,21] The ADNM has not yet been validated in the oncology and palliative care setting.

✔ Tool

Demoralization Scale (DS and DS-II)

Demoralization has been examined by using assessment tools, such as the Demoralization Scale (DS) in its original 24-item version[22] or its more refined 16-item version, DS-II.[23] See Appendix 3.

Recent validation of a short form of the DS showed good sensitivity and specificity as a screening tool for the recognition of demoralization against a diagnostic interview (DCPR) to diagnose clinically significant demoralization.[24] Patients can use a 3-point Likert response (never, sometimes, often) as used in the DS-II, or clinicians can ask patients to rate how much each symptom bothers, concerns, or causes distress on a 11-point visual analog scale, where zero reflects the absence of this symptom and 10 corresponds with the worst possible experience of the symptom.

✔ Tool

Psycho-Existential Symptom Assessment Scale (PeSAS)

Back in 1991, when Bruera and colleagues introduced the original Edmonton Symptom Assessment Scale (ESAS), it included symptoms of anxiety, depression, and family concerns. Many palliative care services have dropped the mental symptoms from the ESAS through lack of confidence in such assessment. The Psycho-Existential Symptom Assessment Scale (PeSAS) has been introduced to reemphasize the importance of assessing such symptoms.[25] See Appendix 4.

Clinicians can build efficacy in screening with the PeSAS through communication skills training, wherein they can practice in simulated role-play scenarios explaining these symptoms to patients. Use of two to three synonyms of any symptom as shown in Box 3.3 helps patient understanding.

Clinical Management

The assessment process will have given you knowledge of the patient's illness severity and prognosis, character strengths that will assist the therapy and any vulnerabilities that could be targets of the treatment. You will be able to plan the length of your intervention proportional to the patient's prognosis. The clinician should be able to summarize the key findings that lead to the diagnosis, empathize with the patient regarding the experience, and see if the patient agrees with the clinician's summary. The clinician can seek permission from the patient to begin a discussion of the potential management plan.

Symptoms occur across three levels of presentation: mild, moderate, and severe. Let us consider management across these three levels. The more severe the symptom profile, the more intensive the therapeutic response needs to be. As shown in Figure 3.1, the management algorithm is tailored to each individual and their family, with continuity of care and length of intervention determined by this severity of presentation.

Box 3.3 Synonyms of Psychoexistential Symptoms

PeSAS Symptoms	Simple Synonyms
Anxiety	Worry, Nervous, Restless
Discouragement	Low morale, disheartened, low confidence
Trapped by illness	Stuck, feeling blocked
Hopelessness	No future, pessimistic
Pointlessness	No meaning, no purpose, no value to life
Loss of control	Helpless, can't plan
Loss of roles	Partner, parent, job, loss of identity or self-worth
Depression	Sad, low mood, no interest, joy, or pleasure
Wish to die	Not go on, want to end it, opposite of wish to live, suicidal
Confusion	Poor memory, disoriented, delirious, confused about things

MANAGEMENT ALGORITHM

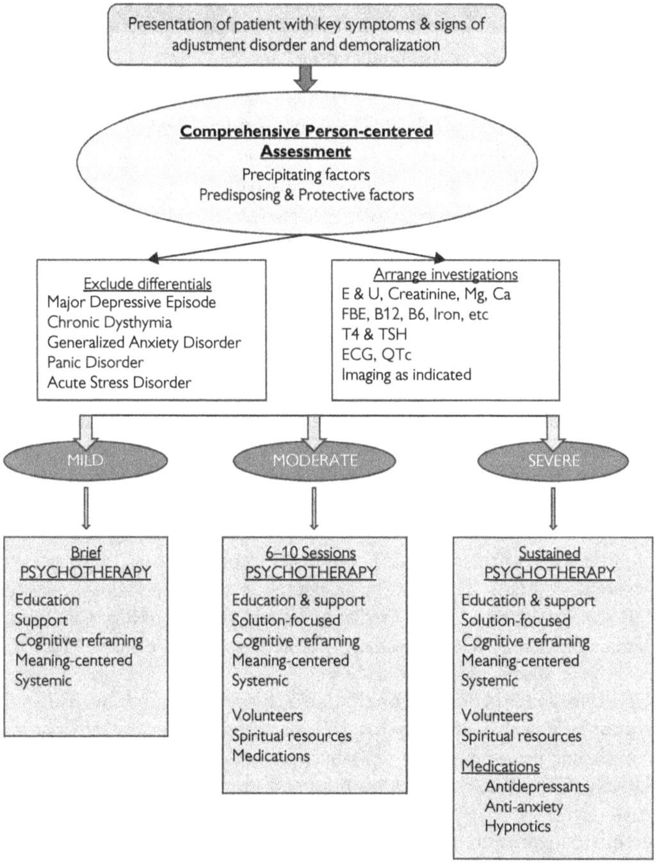

Figure 3.1 Clinical management of adjustment disorder with demoralization is based on the severity of the mental state.

Responding to the Mild Symptom Level

⚲ Key Point

This approach is used when patients express symptoms of low morale, discouragement, and some hopelessness. Clinicians need to understand the circumstances in which these symptoms have developed. What precipitated their onset? Addressing this may be the key to management.

Psychoeducational approach: Can be the starting point for many. The clinician poses questions as illustrated in Box 3.4 and works with the patient to build understanding.

Emotion-focused approach: Follows on from the education above. Here the clinician acknowledges any grief, cautions about the burden of too

> **Box 3.4 Issues to Be Explored in a Psychoeducational Approach**
>
> • How well is the prognosis understood?
> • With whom has grief been shared?
> • What optimizes symptom control? How do you respond to medications?
> • What aspects of your life do you still exercise control over?
> • What brings most sense of purpose to each day?
> • What role brings joy and continuing fulfillment?
> • What relationships matter and can be shared today/this week?
> • Are there aspects of life you are grateful for? People to thank?
> • Any unfinished business? People you want to connect with?

much anticipatory grief, connects the patient to sources of support and offers gentle encouragement about a constructive way forward. Hope is named as a helpful emotion that human beings depend on. Building some focused hope back again can be developed as a therapeutic target.

Meaning-centered approach: The clinician can consider any strengths of character that could be affirmed for this patient. When a patient starts to lose some of their specific hopes in life, people fall back on sources of generalized hope, such as being an optimistic person, perhaps a religious person, having traits of determination and courage, or having what Viktor Frankl termed a "will to meaning." So, what goals and plans will help the person to sustain meaning in their life?

Cognitively oriented approach: Can be built on the above, with identification of negative attitudes that are pessimistic, perhaps catastrophizing, or making use of negative self-labels or predicting the future too negatively. Can these attitudes be reframed in more helpful or constructive terms?

Systemic approach: Could examine the influences of family and friends, who is available for support, and to whom the patient might turn for comfort and support. Is there a relative who also needs a boost? How does the family support one another? Are there unmet needs? Who is a concern? When a clinician reflects upon the contagious nature of demoralization among family and friends, it is immediately evident that a partner or family members may need the clinician's support, as well as or sometimes more so than the patient.

Responding to the Moderate Symptom Level

Again, the clinician needs to understand what precipitated the onset of these symptoms?

 Key Point

This approach is used when there may be predisposing factors in the person, involving a more pessimistic habit in thoughts and attitudes, use of less helpful coping styles or reduced availability of supportive family and friends. In building on the strategies covered above, more attention may be needed to reframe negative cognitions, enhance adaptive coping and foster community supports. Greater continuity of care may be needed, with a program of four to six psychotherapy sessions to foster more adaptive coping, alongside appropriate use of psychotropic medication.

Solution-focused approach: Might examine the benefits or burdens of avoidant versus engaged coping, active versus passive response styles, a doubting versus more trusting approach to relationships, or a worrying versus more confident model of appraisal of challenges. Cognitive reframing may need greater practice to help consolidate improvement.

Meaning-centered approach: Needs to carefully identify strengths of character and lay out the continuity of the person's life story so that accomplishments are better celebrated, the worth of the person is more deeply affirmed, and their connections are engaged with to further validate their creativity and dignity. Only when the clinician can appreciate the rich tapestry of the patient's life journey will sufficient understanding be achieved of whom they are and why they matter.

Volunteers and community supports: Will enrich a patient's support base, provide companionship, ensure respite for the family, and harness the benefits derived from a compassionate community.

Spiritual care: May be needed from chaplaincy and pastoral care services to promote self-acceptance, forgiveness, and connection with the transcendent in their world. Use of ritual and cultural tradition is very helpful (see Chapter 9).

Box 3.5 Issues to Be Explored in Meaning-Centered Therapy

- What key accomplishments from career or roles are you proud of?
- What relationships have brought meaning and fulfilment? Partner? Parent or Grandparent?
- What philosophy of life or religious practice bestows meaning?
- What roles in the community are you proud of?
- What special interest or hobbies foster your creativity?
- Does the experience of music, art, poetry, or literature enrich your life?
- Which friends bring humor, joy, fun, or closeness to you?
- Are there plans, travel, movies, books, or experiences still on your wish list?
- Is there a story, some family history, or an honor you wish to be remembered by?
- Is there a legacy that you wish to leave your descendants?
- Would you like help from a volunteer to record your biography?
- Is there any unfinished business that would place your affairs in good order?

Systemic approach: Delivers support to the patient's partner and/or family members and can be as important for moderate as it was for mild demoralization.

Medication: May prove helpful to allay anxiety, improve sleep, help mood, and support equanimity in the person. Consider hypnotics for sleep, low-dose neuroleptics for anxiety (see Chapter 2), and antidepressants for mood symptoms (see Chapter 4).

As noted in the background section, trials are currently examining the role of psilocybin-assisted therapy for patients with moderate demoralization in the advanced cancer setting. Careful preparation is conducted over three one-hour sessions to prepare eligible patients for psilocybin treatment. They are accompanied over the 6- to 8-hour "trip" brought on by the psychedelic medication with meaningful objects, photographs, and cues positioned around them to introduce and ensure meaning in their experience. They are debriefed over three subsequent 1-hour sessions to make sense of and optimize the meaning found in their experience. The clinical field awaits further trial outcomes to see if this model will be approved by appropriate authorities in each jurisdiction.

Responding to the Severe Symptom Level

🔑 Key Point

This approach is used when symptoms are severe, the likelihood of comorbid mental disorders rises significantly, and so the clinician's assessment of the differential and parallel treatment of any comorbid states becomes paramount. Appropriate use of psychotropic medication for comorbid states is worthwhile.

For demoralization symptoms and those associated with poor adjustment, use is made of psychoeducation, supportive and emotion-focused care, cognitively oriented therapy, meaning-centered therapy, couple and family therapy, and community-based volunteers as described above.

For depressive symptoms, use is made of medications as described in Chapter 4 and for **anxiety symptoms**, use is made of medication as described in Chapter 2.

When coping strategies are maladaptive, counseling that seeks to redirect these into more constructive pathways is paramount. Issues related to communication may benefit from role rehearsal of questions that ought to be asked of other specialists, so that helpful communication is established about the prognosis, goals of care, management of specific physical symptoms, use of prophylactic medications, and supportive care needs. Optimizing instrumental, family and community support is fundamental (see Chapter 7).

Referral of patients in the severe symptom category for psycho-oncology counseling, psychiatric assessment, pastoral care (see Chapter 9) or other specialist allied health support is appropriate with permission.

The Suicidal Patient

When adjustment disorder or demoralization is severe, it is the patient's hopelessness, pointlessness, or worthlessness that generally mediates thoughts that life is no longer worthwhile. A sense of entrapment can be a central symptom that aggravates these states of mind, while poor physical symptom control, un-addressed suffering, unrecognized depression and unabating existential distress can all contribute to the development of suicidal thinking.

In palliative care, as physical frailty develops, acceptance of a person's life coming to a close is normative and needs to be differentiated from suicidal thinking.

The former state of mind involves an awareness of the finitude of life and welcomes natural dying when that occurs. In the latter, a desire to hasten death develops in place of the wish to live, this wish to die being driven by the unpalatability of the quality of life being experienced.

Constant and optimal symptom control is essential to sustain the wish to live.

When the suicidal person develops plans to end their life, urgent management plans ought to include admission to a safe environment, with monitoring by a nursing special, comprehensive assessment, and psychotropic medication to allay agitation and treat depression. Readers could review the chapter "Recognizing and Managing Suicide Risk" in Book 1 of this series.

Case Study (continued)

Team discussion ensured that parenteral nutrition was sustained for Jessica while the trial of cetuximab and encorafenib was provided as anticancer therapy. These goals of care restored hope for Jessica as she set her target on helping her daughter to obtain a dream dress for her Prom. Her CEA tumor markers continued to fall, while imaging revealed regression in the size of her peritoneal nodules. Her morale picked up and she enjoyed valuable family time. Her energy level improved as her serum albumin rose.

Jessica was aware of clinical debate about the wisdom of using TPN and felt blessed to have this opportunity. Supportive therapy sessions continued weekly as she was invited to identify sources of meaning and focus on these. Some flatus returned per rectum for a short while, before disappearing again. Gastroenterology endoscopy and further imaging showed persisting multilevel pressure points on her bowel. Jessica sensed her body was not heading toward a miracle, and indeed after three months of falling CEA levels, they started to rise again. Jessica stayed present centered in her focus, delighting in time with family and friends. She celebrated her daughter's Prom with great delight! She spoke of how the nutritional support restored a sense of control while the immune therapy helped, and yet her overall frailty permitted acceptance that one day life would stop. She sustained her sense of purposeful engagement in activities of deep meaning to her. Her courage was a privilege to watch and support. When abdominal pain worsened, a syringe driver was needed for pain relief and Jessica began to say her goodbyes.

Professional Issues and Service Implementation

Recording and Communicating
To ask a patient about "distress" was promoted as a nonspecific inquiry that was not stigmatized in the manner that attention to their mood with a question

about depression was felt to be. To ask about a person's coping, however, is less directed to mood and more about their way of dealing with or adapting to their predicament or illness. The challenge in an era of patient-reported outcomes measurement information system (PROMIS) medicine has been the focus on symptoms of depression, anxiety, and anger in evaluating mental symptoms, with unspoken assumptions about which mental symptoms are important to monitor. Computer adaptive testing using item response theory started with established questionnaires that focused on mood rather than coping. Such developments have been a statistical triumph on the one hand, yet they may have inadvertently taken the focus away from communicating about other dimensions of the human experience that remain vital.

Where palliative care services have strong usage of physical symptom screens such as the Edmonton Symptom Assessment Scale, screening for psycho-existential symptoms has emerged as a recent focus of activity. As with many symptom assessment programs, unless there is a direct checking for the presence of certain symptoms, they can be avoided for fear of opening the Pandora's box or the clinician fearing they will struggle to respond adequately to this need. The Psycho-existential Symptom Assessment Scale (PeSAS) is one way to screen for, document, and then ensure that multidisciplinary teams attend to existential needs.

Communications skills training programs have much to offer clinicians seeking to build their efficacy in asking about less familiar symptoms like pointlessness, entrapment, or discouragement that are central to constructs such as demoralization.

When a psychosocial assessment as outlined in this chapter has been undertaken, a letter back to the referring clinician that formulates understanding of the patient and their clinical diagnosis can be very helpful, as well as details of planned interventions. Follow-up feedback to the clinical team about ongoing management can occur during multidisciplinary team meetings. Critical changes in patient well-being always necessitate additional communication.

Cultural Issues

The translation of the Demoralization Scale and its subsequent validation into 20 languages provides broad evidence of its cross-cultural validity. Concepts of hope, meaning, and suicidal thinking have universal understanding. The word "morale" might not be as broadly used; for instance, there is no direct translation into Norwegian. The confidence and enthusiasm of a person, the sense of common purpose creating loyalty, commitment, and an esprit de corps to the team or troops, or an individual's psychological well-being with regard to future tasks provide understanding of the word "morale" in its common English use. Synonyms for the word "morale" include "spirit," "self-confidence," "zeal," "assured certainty," and "freedom from doubt," a manner of thinking or resolve that reflects determination and firmness of purpose. According to etymology, the word "demoralize" emerged around the French revolution to describe the loss of morale, courage, hope, and confidence of people undertaking a hazardous enterprise, and was distinguished from morality or ethics. The utility of the word "demoralization" lies in its wide cross-cultural meaning as a construct.

Nevertheless, at the end of life, societies adjust with different customs and traditions. The world's religions offer much guidance about how to face death and what rituals to follow. Due allowance has to be made to such cultural and ethnic variation when assessing coping. Acceptance of the finitude of life may arise from the wisdom of the person, a belief in God's will, confidence in the gentle passage to the next life, or a social expectation to display courage or a stiff upper lip. The art of good clinical practice lies in a sensitive understanding of each patient, their philosophy of life, religious tradition, and cultural influences. Discernment of the normative sadness that one person experiences at the closure of their life from the maladaptive giving up of another is at the heart of this competent and compassionate clinical care provision.

Legal Responsibilities

Clinicians working in palliative care will meet differences in legal access to opioids for pain management, diversion of substances for illicit purposes, or addiction to opioids when used for chronic nonmalignant pain. Each of these predicaments will have substantial impacts on a patient's adjustment and risk of demoralization as a clinical outcome.

Jurisdictions will also differ locally in legislation governing the use of Advance Care Plans (see Chapter 1) at the end of life. Care may be needed when a clinical service is encouraging patient completion of Advance Care Plans that the patient has full mental capacity at such a time. Specific country laws will impact some aspects of care and clinicians need to work within their own country's laws.

Common Ethical Dilemmas

The impact of depression on decision-making at the end of life has implications in jurisdictions that permit medical aid in dying (MAID), euthanasia, or physician-assisted suicide, where a systematic review of 23 studies in medical settings identified a prevalence of impaired decision-making capacity in 34% (95% CI 25%–44%) of clinically depressed patients.[26] In similar manner, severe demoralization may impair a person's ability to appreciate the worth and value of their future, encumber their agency to self-govern and alter their judgment capacity in an ethically important manner.[27] Decision-making capacity warrants careful assessment when demoralization is present.

These issues further impact decisions made by surrogate decision-makers in understanding a person's wishes. **Advance care plans** are promoted as a means to make explicit the values of a person when a medical power of attorney has been issued to a surrogate decision-maker to guide choices when a patient is no longer able to exercise their personal agency and autonomy.

Ethical dilemmas can arise when the needs of a patient sit in tension with the needs of family members at the end of life. Facilitators of family meetings can grapple with such conflicting needs that, in turn, can be compounded by the development of demoralization in either the patient or the family-as-a-whole.

Policies for Clinical Services

Hospice and palliative care have developed from the momentum of visionary clinicians and funders, rather than from national policies funded by governments. Nevertheless, palliative medicine is ahead of many disciplines in using the World Health Organization to foster policy and encourage governments to attend to the care of the dying. Even in countries where healthcare is fully paid for by government, disparities still exist in cancer care with resultant poorer outcomes for citizens who are less educated and socioeconomically deprived. Distress screening has been named as the sixth vital sign in an effort to develop psycho-oncology services across the globe as a basic human right. Policy development is recognized as a basic pathway to generate improved care provision.

The question of recognition of and clinical response to psycho-existential distress at the end of life is a pertinent issue for psycho-oncology services. Policy is needed to ensure that psycho-existential symptoms are screened for and monitored using digitized medical records to ensure that psychosocial issues are addressed alongside physical causes of suffering. Comprehensive medical records are critical to generate data identifying unmet needs and justifying staffing levels by sufficient numbers of psychosocial clinicians to respond to this need.

Teams and Supervision Challenges

Liaison psychiatrists, clinical psychologists, and allied professions play a part in considering the functioning of the multidisciplinary team, ensuring that it operates within a biopsychosocial and spiritual framework rather than following a medical model. Palliative care teams strive to consider the needs of both the patient and their family, including predictions of bereavement risk for care providers. In the face of suffering, where clinical predicaments have involved circumstances of skin breakdown, malodorous wounds, feculent vomiting, unrelenting pain, or unrecognized psycho-existential distress, demoralization can develop not only in patients and their families but also in their treating clinicians and teams-as-a-whole.

🔍 Key Point

The presentation of demoralization in a clinical team takes on the features of burnout, with clinicians displaying exhaustion, detachment, and loss of morale in caring for patients and families. So-called difficult patients and families, where anger, complaints, and demands leave staff feeling criticized, despite their best efforts to care for the sick, create vulnerability for such development.

Palliative care teams use debriefing and routine death review processes to identify such challenges and to ensure the prevention of burnout among team members. Psychosocial staff carry a particular responsibility to monitor such circumstances, provide a deeper understanding of the dynamics of difficult clients, enrich care plans in response to these challenges, and help multidisciplinary teams to sustain their well-being in the face of human suffering and death.

The supervision of psychological and family support staff is a wise principle for services to follow, as these clinicians care for some of the most challenging patients in dire circumstances at the end of life. Universal existential challenges need to be identified and discussed in personal supervision lest avoidance of unresolved issues in the therapist become avoidance of issues in the patient.

References

1. Zelviene P, Kazlauskas E. Adjustment disorder: Current perspectives. Neuropsychiatr Dis Treat. 2018;14:375–381.

2. O'Donnell ML, Agathos JA, Metcalf O, Gibson K, Lau W. Adjustment disorder: Current developments and future directions. Int J Environ Res Public Health. 2019;16(14):2537.

3. Kissane DW. Demoralization—A life-preserving diagnosis to make in the severely medically ill. J Palliat Care. 2014;30(4):255–258.

4. Mitchell AJ, Chan M, Bhatti H, et al. Prevalence of depression, anxiety, and adjustment disorder in oncological, haematological, and palliative-care settings: A meta-analysis of 94 interview-based studies. Lancet Oncol. 2011;12:160–174.

5. Robinson S, Kissane, DW, Brooker, J, Burney, S. A systematic review of the demoralization syndrome in individuals with progressive disease and cancer: A decade of research. J Pain Sympt Manage. 2015;49(3):595–610. http://dx.doi.org/10.1016/j.jpainsymman.2014.07.008.

6. Tecuta L, Tomba E, Grandi S, Fava GA. Demoralization: A systematic review on its clinical characterization. Psych Med. 2015;45(4):673–691.

7. Tang PL, Wang HH, Chou FH. A systematic review and meta-analysis of demoralisation and depression in patients with cancer. Psychosom. 2015;56(6):634–643.

8. Bachem R, Casey P. Adjustment disorder: A diagnosis whose time has come. J Affect Dis. 2018;227:243–253.

9. Kazlauskas E, Zelviene P, Lorenz L, Quero S, Maercker A. A scoping review of ICD-11 adjustment disorder research. Eur J Psychotraumatol. 2018;8(sup7):1 421819.

10. Maercker A, Lorenz L. Adjustment disorder diagnosis: Improving clinical utility. World J Biol Psychiatry. 2018;19(sup1):S3–S13.

11. Guidi J, Fava GA, Picardi A, et al. Subtyping depression in the medically ill by cluster analysis. J Affect Dis. 2011;132(3):383–388

12. Bobevski I, Kissane DW, Vehling S, McKenzie D, Glaesmer H, Mehnert A. Latent class analysis differentiation of adjustment disorder and demoralization, more severe depressive-anxiety disorders, and somatic symptoms in a cohort of patients with cancer. Psycho-Oncology. 2018;27(11):2623–2630, https://doi.org/10.1002/pon.4761.

13. Belvederi Murri M, Caruso R, Ounalli H, et al. The relationship between demoralization and depressive symptoms among patients from the general hospital: Network and exploratory graph analysis. J Affective Dis. 2020;276:137–146. https://doi.org/10.1016/j.jad.2020.06.074

14. Breitbart W, Pessin H, Rosenfeld B, et al. Individual meaning-centered psychotherapy for the treatment of psychological and existential distress: A randomized controlled trial in patients with advanced cancer. Cancer. 2018;124(15):3231–3239. https://doi.org/10.1002/cncr.31539.

15. Rodin G, Lo C, Rydall A, et al. Managing Cancer and Living Meaningfully (CALM): A randomized controlled trial of a psychological intervention for

patients with advanced cancer. J Clin Oncol. 2018;36(23):2422–2432. https://doi.org/10.1200/JCO.2017.77.1097.

16. Ross S, A Bossis, Guss J, et al. Rapid and sustained symptom reduction following psilocybin treatment for anxiety and depression in patients with life-threatening cancer: A randomized controlled trial. J Psychopharm. 2016;30(12):1165–1180. https://doi.org/10.1177/0269881116675512.

17. Anderson BT, Danforth A, Daroff R, et al. Psilocybin-assisted group therapy for demoralized older long-term AIDS survivor men: An open-label safety and feasibility pilot study. E Clin Med. 2020; https://doi.org/10.1016/j.eclinm.2020.100538.

18. Bachem R, Perkonigg A, Stein DJ, Maercker A. Measuring the ICD-11 adjustment disorder concept: Validity and sensitivity to change of the Adjustment Disorder—New Module questionnaire in a clinical intervention study. Int J Methods Psychiatr Res. 2017;26(4):e1545.

19. Liang L, Ben-Ezra M, Chan EWW, Liu H, Lavenda O, Hou WK. Psychometric evaluation of the Adjustment Disorder New Module-20 (ADNM-20): A multistudy analysis. J Anxiety Disord. 2021;81:102406. https://doi.org/10.1016/j.janxdis.2021.102406..

20. Ben-Ezra M, Mahat-Shamir M, Lorenz L, Lavenda O, Maercker A. Screening of adjustment disorder: Scale based on the ICD-11 and the Adjustment Disorder New Module. J Psychiatr Res. 2018;103:91–96.

21. Lavenda O, Mahat-Shamir M, Lorenz L, et al. Revalidation of Adjustment Disorder-New Module-4 screening of adjustment disorder in a non-clinical sample: Psychometric reevaluation and correlates with other ICD-11 mental disorders Psych J. 2019;8(3):378–385.

22. Kissane DW, Wein S, Love A, Lee XQ, Kee PL, Clarke DM. The Demoralization Scale: A preliminary report of its development and preliminary validation. J Palliat Care. 2004;20(4):269–276.

23. Robinson S, Kissane DW, Brooker J, et al. Refinement and revalidation of the Demoralization Scale: The DS-II—internal validity. Cancer. 2016;122:2251–2259. https://doi.org/10.1002/cncr.30015.

24. Belvederi Murri M, Zerbinatia L, Ounalli H, et al. Assessing demoralisation in medically ill patients: Factor structure of the Italian version of the demoralisation scale and development of short versions with the item response theory framework. J Psychosom Res. 2020;128:109889. https://doi.org/10.1016/j.jpsychores.2019.109889..

25. Kissane DW. Education and assessment of psycho-existential symptoms to prevent suicidality in cancer care. Psycho-Oncology. 2020;29(9). https://doi.org/10.1002/pon.5519website seems to be working well.

26. Lepping P, Stanly T, Turner J. Systematic review on the prevalence of lack of capacity in medical and psychiatric settings. Clin Med (London). 2015;15(4):337–343. https://doi.org/10.7861/clinmedicine.15-4-337.

27. Mendz GL, Kissane DW. Agency, autonomy and euthanasia. J Law Med Ethics. 2020;48:555–564. https://doi.org/10.1177/1073110520958881

Further Reading

Breitbart W, Poppito SR. Individual Meaning-Centered Psychotherapy for Patients with Advanced Cancer: A Treatment Manual. New York: Oxford University Press; 2014. A definitive guide to conducting meaning-centered therapy for palliative care patients.

Chochinov HM, Breitbart W, Editors. Handbook of Psychiatry in Palliative Medicine. 3rd ed. New York: Oxford University Press; 2022. This is the leading textbook at the interface of psychiatry, psychology, and palliative care. It offers a more detailed coverage of the diagnosis and management of issues covered in this chapter.

Grassi L, Riba M, Wise T, Editors. Person Centered Approach to Recovery in Medicine. Cham, Switzerland: Springer, 2019. This book proposes integration methods in screening and assessment, a clinimetric approach, dignity conserving care, and cross-cultural and ethical aspects as well as treatment and training.

Casey P, Editor. Adjustment Disorder: From Controversy to Clinical Practice. 1st ed. Oxford: Oxford University Press; 2018. The volume provides concise and comprehensive information on Adjustment Disorders.

Chapter 4

Depressive Disorders

Daisuke Fujisawa, Tatsuo Akechi, and Yosuke Uchitomi

Learning Objectives

After reading this chapter, the clinician will be able to:

1. Understand the signs and symptoms of clinical depression in palliative care practice.
2. Conduct a comprehensive assessment, excluding differential diagnoses and assessing the psychosocial needs of patients with advanced cancer.
3. Understand the basic principles of treatment, including use of psychotropic medication and psychotherapy.
4. Make a referral to a specialist when appropriate.
5. Describe ethical, cultural, legal, and professional issues that may arise in the clinical care of patients with depression in the palliative and end of life (EOL) context.

Background Evidence

Depression, which is characterized by depressed mood and/or loss of interest and pleasure, is a common syndrome among patients with life-threatening illness. The prevalence of depression and depressive disorders among patients with cancer is between 5% and 60% according to the different diagnostic criteria, different stages, and types of cancer.[1] The prevalence of major depression among cancer patients according to stringent criteria is 16.3% (13.4%–19.5%), with another 19.2% (9.1%–31.9%) suffering from minor depression (a milder type of depression).[2] Patients with more advanced illness have a higher prevalence of depression, and in the former meta-analysis, prevalence of any mood disorder was 29% in palliative care settings. In a recent meta-analysis of 15 good-quality psychiatric interview-based studies, the prevalence of depression was reported to vary from 7% to 49% in palliative care patients.[3] The data of a further systematic review of 59 studies conducted in several settings (e.g., hospital departments, oncology departments, hospice/palliative care units, and outpatient services) showed a 2%–56% prevalence of depression.[4] These figures are two to three times higher than those of the general population and similar to what are found in patients with other physical illness.[5]

Depression not only causes suffering for patients, it also impairs patients' well-being in many ways. Even a mild level of depression can cause significant decrements in quality of life, which is comparable to decrements due to major physical symptom burden and decreased performance status.[6] Depression is associated with poorer health outcomes and shorter survival in cancer patients, due to both death by cancer and death by other causes.[7,8] Lower survival of patients with depression is partly explained by poorer adherence to cancer treatment,[9] poorer self-care (e.g., unfavorable lifestyle such as decreased level of physical exercise, higher alcohol consumption, or inappropriate diet), and proneness to medical decisions that may shorten life (e.g., receiving chemotherapy at the very end of life, which can do more harm than good regarding survival).[10] There is some evidence that depression decreases immune function, although its relationship with cancer prognosis remains unclear.[11] In clinical management, patients with depression tend to stay longer in hospitals. Depression often increases sensitivity to and monitoring of physical sensations and thereby may increase pain. Also, depression can influence patients' decision-making capacity.[12] Depression is a large contributor to the wish for hastened death (e.g., suicide, physician-assisted suicide, euthanasia, and rejection of proper treatment).[13]

Both biological and psychosocial factors are involved in depression. Recently, mounting evidence indicates that inflammatory cytokines contribute to the development of depression in both medically ill and medically healthy individuals. Chronic exposure to elevated inflammatory cytokines and persistent alterations in neurotransmitter systems can lead to neuropsychiatric disorders such as depression. Mechanisms of cytokine behavioral effects involve activation of inflammatory signaling pathways in the brain that results in changes in monoamine, glutamate, and neuropeptide systems, and decreases in brain-derived growth factor (BDNF).[14]

For cancer patients in particular, some researchers propose that depressive disorders can be categorized into inflammatory depressions and noninflammatory depressions. The former accompanies increased level of inflammation and pro-inflammatory cytokines (such as C-reactive protein (CRP), tumor necrosis factor-alpha (TNF-alpha), interleukin-6 (IL-6), and IL-1beta. These "inflammatory depressions" overlap with the symptoms of "sickness syndrome," which is a pathophysiologic syndrome in medically ill patients that arises within the context of chronic immune activation, and often responds better to dopaminergic antidepressants than other classes of antidepressants.[15]

Depression is frequently underrecognized and undertreated. Severe depression is more likely to be underrecognized since patients with severe depression tend to express their emotions less than those with milder depression. Therefore, routine screening is considered vital in oncology practice.[16]

Meta-analyses provide sound evidence for the effectiveness of antidepressants in the treatment of depression in the cancer setting.[17,18] Similarly, strong evidence is emerging for the role of psychotherapy, including among patients with advanced cancer.[19,20] Reviews confirm the benefits of psychostimulants and ketamine,[21,22] while studies of psilocybin-assisted psychotherapy are starting to show promise, but the evidence for this intervention is not yet robust. Mindfulness-based psychotherapies and a range of complementary therapies are also employed in palliative care.[23] Finally, technology-based and online therapies are beginning to make their contribution.[24,25]

Presenting Problems

Key Symptoms and Signs

Depression is a syndrome characterized by depressed mood and anhedonia (decreased interest or diminished sense of pleasure). It is a spectrum of symptoms, where normal sadness or grief occurs at the milder end and major depression at the opposite (more severe) end. Minor or subthreshold depression lies in the middle.

Major depression is a diagnostic category characterized by five or more (out of nine) depressive symptoms present for most of the day for at least 2 weeks. At least one of those five symptoms must be depressed mood or anhedonia. The other symptoms include decreased energy, remarkable change in appetite (decrease or increase of appetite, which can be allied with change in body weight), sleep disturbance (either insomnia or hypersomnia), psychomotor agitation or retardation (i.e., patients may objectively look irritable or slow in actions), feelings of worthlessness or guilt, difficulty concentrating, and suicidal ideation (see Box 4.1).

A patient is diagnosed as having minor (or subthreshold) depression when two to four of these symptoms are present for at least 2 weeks. A state whereby three to four depressive symptoms are present continuously for at least 2 years is called dysthymia (chronic depression). Although minor depression is described as a milder form of depression, it is associated with

---

Box 4.1 Symptomatology of Major Depressive Disorder

1. Depressed mood
2. Anhedonia (lack of interest or pleasure in almost all activities)
3. Sleep disorder (insomnia or hypersomnia)
4. Appetite loss, weight loss; appetite gain, weight gain
5. Fatigue or loss of energy
6. Psychomotor retardation (patient looks slow in thoughts, actions or responses) or agitation (patient looks irritable and hasty)
7. Trouble concentrating or trouble making decisions
8. Low self-esteem or feelings of guilt
9. Recurrent thoughts of death or suicidal ideation

Five symptoms from the above are required to make the diagnosis of depression and must include depressed mood and/or anhedonia (1.2.).

Note: The symptoms must have been present most of the day, nearly every day for at least two weeks. The symptoms cannot be explained by other physical or psychiatric problems.
Adapted from Diagnostic and Statistical Manual of Mental Disorders, Fifth Edition (DSM-5), American Psychiatric Association, 2013.

significant impairment of quality of life and can be critical, especially among vulnerable populations such as older people or those with poor socioeconomic status. The diagnostic term "adjustment disorder" is often used for milder forms of depression. It refers to a state of moderate to marked distress that is greater than expected from exposure to a stressor and may present with depressive symptoms (see Chapter 3 for details of adjustment disorder). It is of note, especially in oncology and palliative-care settings, that although life stressors may seem to provide "good reasons" for sadness, the diagnosis of depression should be given if a patient meets the criteria for major/minor depression. Supporting symptoms of depressive disorders (and not nonpathological emotional reactions to stressful events) include more pervasive symptoms of depression, loss of emotional reactivity to good news (e.g., a patient who does not feel joy in response to hospital visits of close family), irrational sense of self-guilt (e.g., patients who believe it is their fault they have cancer), and suicidal thoughts, including specific plans. In addition, depressed patients often have physical symptoms (so-called neurovegetative symptoms), such as sleep disturbance, psychomotor retardation, appetite disturbance, poor concentration, and low energy, which can co-occur and/ or mimic the consequences of their underlying illness or treatment, making the diagnosis of depression more difficult in patients receiving palliative and end of life care.

Making a Formal Diagnosis

The diagnosis of depression needs to be made by clinical interviews according to the criterion of either the Diagnostic and Statistical Manual of Mental Disorders 5th edition (DSM-5) or the International Classification of Diseases, 11th edition (ICD-11). Formally, clinicians may refer to a manual of the Structured Clinical Interview for the DSM-5, while in actual clinical practice, clinicians usually simply ask whether a patient has each symptom of depression according to DSM-5 or ICD-11. Clinicians start by asking about the core symptoms of depression (depressive mood and anhedonia). The presence of either of these two symptoms ought to prompt clinicians to perform a full diagnostic assessment of major depression.

The US Preventive Services Task Force recommends the following two-item screening for major depression, although the sensitivity and specificity of such ultrashort screening questions may be limited in palliative care settings:

1. "Over the past two weeks, have you ever felt down, depressed, or hopeless?"
2. "Over the past two weeks, have you felt little interest or pleasure doing things?

Issues Surrounding the Diagnosing of Depression

A difficult issue in diagnosing depression in patients with cancer is that many symptoms of depression, such as appetite loss, weight loss, insomnia, cognitive impairment, fatigue, and energy loss, may be a consequence of cancer or cancer treatment rather than depression. Therefore, there have been debates regarding the need to modify the DSM criteria of major depression when applied to cancer. Several proposals have been suggested, namely: to include all the symptoms irrespective of the fact that these symptoms may or may not be attributable to cancer (inclusive approach), to replace somatic symptoms with cognitive-affective items (substitutive approach), to add some new affective symptoms to the original criteria (alternative approach), and to exclude somatic symptoms and use only affective symptoms to make the diagnosis (exclusive approach).[26] In a recent study involving 969 patients with advanced cancer within the European Palliative Care Research Collaborative-Computer Symptom Assessment Study (EPCRC-CSA), it was shown that the scoring-method, not excluding somatic symptoms, had the greatest effect on assessment outcomes, since depression was significantly associated with pain and lower performance status.[27]

Screening Tools for Depression

Self-administered instruments can serve as screening tools and diagnostic aids for depression, although they cannot substitute for clinical interviews. Short screening tools are easy for patients to administer, however, their specificity in diagnosing depression tends to be low, thus they should be followed by further clinical assessments. The instruments that are widely used in oncology and palliative-care settings[28] include, but are not limited to, the following:

• Distress Thermometer (DT)

The DT is an 11-point numeric scale that mimics a thermometer to self-rate one's distress. The NCCN guidelines recommend a distress score of 4 of 10 as a cutoff. Some modified versions of the DT, such as the Distress and Impact Thermometer (DIT), are also used as a screening tool in some countries, although utility and cutoff scores in patients at end of life stage have not been established.

• Edmonton Symptom Assessment System (ESAS)

The ESAS is a 10-item screening instrument with 11-point numeric scales to detect common physical and psychological symptoms in palliative care settings. The instrument contains one item on depression and one item on anxiety. In a study which enrolled 1,215 cancer patients, a cut-off of ≥2 on the ESAS-Depression item demonstrated a sensitivity of 0.86, specificity of 0.72, positive predictive value of 0.46 and negative predictive value of 0.95.

• Patient Health Questionnaire (PHQ-9 and PHQ-2)

The PHQ-9 is a screening questionnaire that comprises nine questions that correspond to symptoms of DSM-5 major depression. It is a recommended scale by the American Society of Clinical Oncology. A score of 10 or higher has been demonstrated to have 88% sensitivity and 88% specificity for the diagnosis of major depression. Some items (such as tiredness and appetite loss) can be problematic because they may be influenced by the symptoms of advanced cancer and its treatment.

The PHQ-2 is a two-item questionnaire that extracted two core symptoms of depression (depressed mood and anhedonia) from the PHQ-9. It may serve as an ultrashort screener for depression.

- Hospital Anxiety and Depression Scale (HADS)

The HADS is a 14-item self-rating questionnaire that enquires about symptoms of depression and anxiety (seven items each). It is the most widely used measure for depression in oncology settings. Since it does not include somatic symptoms, it eliminates the influence of physical conditions. The most commonly used threshold to define depression is a subscale score of 11 or above (8–10 as "borderline"), although variability in recommended cutoff scores (ranging from 4 to 11) has been reported.

- Beck Depression Inventory (BDI)

The classic BDI and its variations (the BDI-II and the BDI-Short Form [BDI-SF]) are often considered the "gold standard" scales for depression. The limitations include the length (21 items), which can reduce acceptability, and its inclusion of somatic symptoms; the BDI-SF removes physical symptoms and has obvious benefits in oncology practice. The scores 0–3 on BDI-SF indicate minimal depression; 4–6 indicate mild depression; 7–9 indicate moderate depression; and 10–21 indicate severe depression.

Key Problems Associated with Development of Depression

Depression can occur in patients with any type of cancer and at any stage of illness. Key risk factors for depression include:

- past history of depression or other psychiatric disorders
- family history of depression
- advanced illness
- higher symptom burden (e.g., pain)
- more frequent unmet needs (e.g., physical, social, psychological and spiritual)
- high level of inflammatory cytokines (inflammatory depressions)
- use of steroids or other medications associated with depression

Case Study

A 60-year-old male with a diagnosis of advanced lung cancer, with bone and liver metastases, was referred to a psycho-oncologist. The reasons for referral were his wish for hastened death, refusal of treatment with third-line chemotherapy, and his persistent concern about physical symptoms, which were not explained well by physical examination and imaging. Close interview revealed persistent depressive mood, lack of appetite, poor sleep, and excessive fatigue that could not be explained satisfactorily by his physical condition, as well as a lack of motivation toward anything. The patient was diagnosed as having major depression, and mirtazapine 7.5 mg (before sleep) was started. His sleep improved immediately, and his appetite began to pick up after a few days. Although the patient's mood improved a bit and his physical complaints diminished, he was hesitant to get out of his bed because he felt "too fatigued to move." In collaboration with the psycho-oncology and rehabilitation teams, the patient was encouraged to gradually increase his activity level, based on the principles of behavioral activation (see later sections for detail). The patient, his family, and the nurses created an activity schedule, which initially included small activities and later increased activity. Also, elaborate conversations with the patient revealed that his unwillingness to get up arose from a fear of falling and breaking his bones. Followed by the assessment of the interdisciplinary team and reassurance from the treating physician, the patient became more active after a week and started participating in rehabilitation. Although some anxiety about discharge was observable, the primary care team coordinated his discharge after a "trial" of an overnight stay at home, which helped reassure him about his recovery.

Investigations for Key Differential Diagnoses

Key Differentials

Key differentials for depression include unsolved physical symptoms, physical conditions that lead to lowered mood and activities, organic brain disorders and altered mental status (such as delirium), psychiatric illnesses other than depression, and adverse effects of medications (see Box 4.2).

Essential Tests

The potential tests for the differential diagnoses of depression include the following (see Box 4.3). However, clinicians should judiciously select according to the patients' physical condition and available treatments. For example, neuroimaging may not be indicated for patients who are at the end of life, since there would be scarce prospect of successful treatment for organic brain disorders at that stage of illness, and neuroimaging can be a burden for patients who are very sick.

Further Assessments

Depression can be masked, and diagnosis and evaluation of depression cannot occur without clinical interviews. Some patients, especially older patients and those with severe depressive symptoms, may not explicitly admit to lowered mood, which can make the assessment difficult.

🔍 Key Points

The following objective appearance and behaviors of patients may be signs of depression.

- Social withdrawal
- Not participating in medical care
- Diminished positive emotional reactions (e.g., not able to be cheered up, does not smile, no response to good news, visitors, or funny situations)
- Demeanor showing reduced facial reactivity and slowed thinking
- Wish for hastened death

Box 4.2 Key Differential Diagnoses for Depression

Physical Conditions
- Unsolved physical distress (e.g., pain, nausea)
- Endocrine dysfunction (e.g., hyperthyroidism, hypothyroidism, adrenal insufficiency), which can be caused by either surgical resection, radiation therapy, immune therapies, or cancer metastases.
- Anemia
- Diabetes mellitus
- Nutritional deficiency (vitamin B3 [nicotinic acid, niacin], vitamin B12, folate, vitamin C)
- Electrolyte imbalance (sodium, potassium, calcium, magnesium)
- Certain cancers causing cytokine cascades (CRP, low albumin)
- Cancer-related fatigue
- Other exhausting physical conditions, such as cardiac dysfunction, hepatic dysfunction, infection, pulmonary dysfunction

Organic Brain Disorders
- Cancer-related
  - Brain tumor or metastasis, especially frontal lobe apathy
  - Meningitis carcinomatosis, or leptomeningeal disease
  - Paraneoplastic syndrome
- Other neurological disorders
  - Parkinson's syndrome, multiple sclerosis, HIV encephalopathy, cerebrovascular diseases, etc.
- Changed mental status
  - Consciousness disturbance, including delirium (especially hypoactive delirium)

Other Psychiatric/Psychological States
- Alcohol/substance abuse (chronic alcohol abuse can cause depressive symptoms, which can be alleviated by abstinence)
- Normal grief (normal psychological reaction to stress)
- Demoralization syndrome (see chapter 3)

Medications (Side Effects)
- Steroids, interferon, beta-adrenergic blockers, calcium-channel blockers, benzodiazepines, barbiturates, cholinergic medications, estrogens
- Late effect of anticancer agents ("chemobrain")

Medications (Withdrawal)
- Steroids
- Stimulants

Box 4.3 Essential Tests for Diagnosing Major Depression

- Laboratory tests to exclude:
  - Anemia (Hb, Ht)
  - Electrolyte disturbance (Na, K, Ca, Mg)
  - Hypoglycaemia (Glu)
  - Endocrine disorders (thyroid tests [TSH, fT3, fT4], ACTH, cortisol)
  - Liver function tests if metastatic liver disease
  - C-Reactive Protein
  - albumin
  - Electroencephalogram (EEG): when consciousness disturbance is suspected
  - Neuroimaging: CT brain scan, MRI brain (Gd-enhancement is recommended to detect subtle brain metastasis, leptomeningeal disease, or meningitis carcinomatosis)

Factors That Contribute to Misdiagnosis or Inappropriate Care

Fatigue and devastating physical conditions

Devastating physical consequences from cancer and its treatment can mimic depressive symptoms. For example, poor appetite, weight loss, and fatigue can be symptoms due to cancer (and cancer treatments) or depression (see Table 4.1). This dilemma is commonly found in a patient with severe cancer cachexia. Fatigue and depression are differentiated by assessing the presence of depressive mood or anhedonia. In cases of uncertainty, an empirical trial of antidepressant therapy may be worthwhile to ensure that a possible patient with depression does not go untreated.

Table 4.1 Distinguishing Fatigue from Depression

Clinical State	Key Features
Fatigue	• Patients are usually able to derive some pleasure from activities that they normally find enjoyable.
	• Late afternoon is the most difficult time of the day.
	• Higher prevalence than depression.
Depression	• Patients are unable to experience pleasure from experiences that they usually enjoy.
	• Morning is the most difficult time of the day.
	• Patients may have suicidal thoughts and hopelessness (Pt with fatigue may also).
	• Prior history and/or family history of depression may increase the likelihood of developing an episode of depression.
Prior history	• These may increase the likelihood of developing an episode of depression.
Family history	• Caveat: fatigue and depression may be concurrent.

🔍 Key Point

The rule of thumb is to diagnose a patient as depressed and offer a therapeutic trial of treatment unless there is clear evidence that his or her depressive symptoms come from physical issues. This avoids missing the chance to help the patient recover from depression (inclusive approach).

✓ Tool

Exemplary diagnostic questions include the following:

1. "Do you feel depressed all the time? Or do you feel better when your physical symptoms are relatively better?" (If a patient replies "yes" to the latter question, he or she probably does not have a depressive mood symptom).
2. "Are you motivated to do something if your physical symptoms are relieved?" (If a patient replies "yes" to this question, he or she is probably not anhedonic).
3. "If you weren't so fatigued, do you think you'd still be depressed?"

Delirium

Delirium, especially hypoactive delirium, is often misdiagnosed as depression (or vice versa). Common symptoms between delirium (especially mild-level delirium) and depression include decreased level of motivation and/or activity, decreased level of emotional reactions and psychomotor retardation. Also, irritability may be found in both diagnoses. See Chapter 5 for the assessment of delirium.

Clinical Management

The overview of clinical management of depression is shown in Figure 4.1. The clinical approach to depression begins with routine screening, followed by detailed assessment and appropriate treatment according to the severity of depression.

Screening and Referral

Routine screening for psychological distress (including depression) is necessary, especially at critical time points of cancer care (e.g., after receiving some "bad news," during transition from one treatment modality to another). Following such screening, comprehensive assessment and support should be provided.

Good Communication and Proactive Need Assessments

Good communication between clinicians and patients is fundamental to preventing and alleviating depression. For example, providing communication skill training to oncologists can result in a decrease of psychological distress among their patients. Proactive, detailed assessment and addressing patients' needs and concerns are important components of psychosocial care. In this

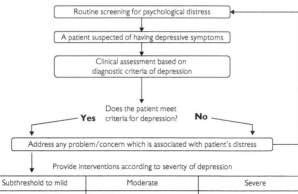

Figure 4.1 Clinical assessment and management of a patient with depression.

regard, provision of palliative care that is integrated into routine oncology practice from an earlier stage of treatment for advanced lung cancer patients has been shown to alleviate depression without increasing referral to mental health specialists.

Treatment

Although there is substantial evidence regarding treatment of depression in patients with cancer, there has been no solid evidence in palliative and end of life care settings since clinical trials have been scarce in this population. Thus, here we first present the principles of treatment of depression in general oncology practice, then we refer to a few issues to be considered in palliative care and end of life care.

Two major treatment modalities of depression are psychotherapy and pharmacotherapy. Their indications are considered based on patients' preference, their physical condition, depression severity, and access to care. Psychotherapy (psychological treatment) is indicated for all levels of depression severity, but usually preferred in milder cases, since it takes a longer time before it becomes effective. Its advantage over pharmacotherapy is its relapse-prevention effect, which means that the effect of psychotherapy is sustained after the treatment has stopped. Pharmacotherapy usually takes a shorter time to be effective than psychotherapy, and its effect size is larger in more severe than in mild cases. Therefore, it is considered a requirement for severe depression and an option for mild to moderate depression. In palliative and end of life care settings, special consideration should be given regarding the patients' physical condition and prognosis, as the predicted length of time impacts greatly on the selection of treatment toward the end of life. Sometimes, the patients' vulnerable physical condition may limit the use of pharmacotherapy; at the same time, certain types of psychotherapy would be too lengthy to complete.

Psychotherapy (Psychological Treatments)

General Principles

There is robust evidence supporting psychological treatments for patients with cancer, and a variety of techniques and methods have been developed and examined for their effectiveness in the psychological care of cancer patients, which will be described later. Before implementing a psychotherapeutic strategy, it is important to develop a formulation and to consider whether the patient is eligible for psychotherapy, what type of psychotherapy is most suitable, and what the patient's preferences are regarding treatment approach. Generally, implementation of psychotherapy requires that patients are highly motivated and that symptoms of clinical depression do not represent a barrier to patients' abilities to use talking therapies.

Relaxation Techniques

Relaxation techniques are a widely used method in the field of oncology. Meta-analyses demonstrate effectiveness for various physical and psychological conditions, including depression, anxiety, breathlessness, and pain, although efficacy appears to be short-lived. Three typical techniques are: (1) progressive muscle relaxation, (2) breathing techniques, and (3) imagery (autoinduction techniques). The evidence indicates this method is more helpful for the management of anxiety than depression. Relaxation techniques are often used as a part of a more structured program of psychotherapy (such as cognitive-behavioral therapy [CBT] and problem-solving therapy [PST]).

Cognitive-Behavioral Therapy

Cognitive-behavioral therapy, or cognitive therapy, is a structured psychotherapy based on the hypothesis that one's emotional and somatic responses (mood and physical symptoms) are determined by how one perceives a situation, rather than the situation itself. CBT primarily involves identifying and correcting inaccurate or dysfunctional thoughts and behaviors associated with negative feelings (e.g., depression and/or anxiety) and distressing physical symptoms (e.g., pain, fatigue), practicing relaxation techniques and enhancing problem-solving skills. A fuller explanation of CBT can be found in the Handbook of Psychotherapy in Cancer Care (see Further Reading). Behavioral activation (BA), an intervention rooted in CBT, has also been shown to decrease depression in patients with cancer. The hypothesis of BA is that people who are depressed are trapped in the vicious cycle of feeling depressed—loss of energy (loss of motivation)—loss of opportunities for feeling pleasure or sense of achievement—feeling more depressed. The therapist encourages patients to undertake activities that bring them pleasure or feelings of achievement by encouraging them to develop a schedule of daily activities and monitor mood changes that result from each activity. There is robust evidence that CBT and BA are effective for patients with cancer with a reasonable prognosis (e.g., several weeks or longer); however, it becomes less relevant when patients are close to the end of life (see also Chapter 2).

Problem-Solving Therapy

Problem-solving therapy is often described as a simpler or more focused form of CBT and is based on the hypothesis that psychological distress is linked with unsolved problems; therefore, acquisition of efficient problem-solving (or coping) leads to decreased distress. In the standard problem-solving therapy procedure, the therapist teaches methods of efficacious problem-solving, which is achieved through: (1) defining the problem, (2) brainstorming possible options, (3) evaluating potential solutions by weighing the advantages and disadvantages of each solution, (4) implementing specific solutions, (5) evaluating their degree of success, and (6) fine-tuning them. Since this is a quite straightforward method, it can be implemented by health professionals who are not specialized in mental health (e.g., primary care nurses) and who have been through a relatively short training.

Supportive Psychotherapy

Supportive psychotherapy encourages patients to verbalize their emotions and supports them in pursuit of their personal goals. Several types of supportive psychotherapy have been evaluated in clinical trials among patients with cancer. Compared with CBT, supportive psychotherapies have been more widely tested for patients with advanced cancers.

Meaning-Centered Psychotherapy

Meaning-centered psychotherapy (MCP) is an eight-week manualized intervention that can be delivered in either an individual or a group format. The intervention is based on the work of Viktor Frankl's logotherapy and aims to help patients with advanced cancer sustain or enhance a sense of meaning in their lives. Each session addresses specific themes related to an exploration of the concepts and sources of meaning (e.g., historical [i.e., legacy], attitudinal, creative, and experiential sources of meaning).

Dignity Therapy

Dignity therapy (DT) is a brief individual therapy designed to address existential distress in patients near the end of life. Dignity, a fundamental of one's psychological well-being, is considered to include themes of generativity and continuity of self, maintenance of pride and hope, role preservation, alleviation of concerns about being a burden to others, and the aftermath of his or her death. The typical initial prompt of a dignity-therapy counselor is: *"Tell me a little about your life history, particularly the parts that you either remember most or think were most important."* The goal is to elicit the aspects of the patient's life that he or she considers meaningful or that he or she wants to be remembered for. The conversation between the patient and the therapist is tape-recorded, transcribed, edited, and passed on to the patient as a "generativity document," which can be shared with family.

Managing Cancer and Living Meaningfully (CALM) Therapy

The managing cancer and living meaningfully (CALM) therapy is a brief psychotherapy, which is designed to address specific problems that may be associated with psychological distress as well as psychological growth of patients with advanced cancer. It consists of four empirically derived domains of concern: (1) symptom management and communication with healthcare providers; (2) changes in self and relations with close others; (3) spirituality or sense of meaning and purpose; and (4) thinking of the future, hope, and mortality.

Interpersonal Psychotherapy

Interpersonal psychotherapy (IPT) has been proven to be as efficacious as CBT for alleviating depression, although it has not been well studied in oncology settings. IPT hypothesizes that depression can arise from unsolved issues with people's significant others (i.e., people who are close to them), usually in any of the following four realms: grief, disputes, role transitions, and lack of significant relationships. IPT therapists try to identify the interpersonal problems of the patient and to solve them through various techniques, including cognitive behavioral skills, and communication analysis and training.

Family and Couple Therapy

A cancer diagnosis can cause distress in partners and family members of patients with cancer; thus, interventions aiming at both patients and their families together may be more efficacious than aiming at an individual. Couple therapy aims to enhance relationships and to protect patients and their partners against relational distress. The rationale of couple therapist is that the needs, goals, and coping responses of patients and their partners are highly correlated and reciprocally interdependent. It has been widely studied among breast and prostate cancer populations. Poor family function is associated with higher relapse rates of depression and the development of complicated grief. Family therapy, which aims to optimize family functioning through promotion of effective communication, enhanced cohesion, and adaptive resolution of conflict, has been shown to reduce depression and support mourning after family loss due to cancer among low-functioning families.

Pharmacotherapy

General Principles

Antidepressants are the first-choice drugs for adult depression (see Table 4.2). This also applies to depressed patients who have comorbid cancer, although further clinical trials in this population are needed to draw firm conclusions. In palliative and end of life care settings, psychotropics other than antidepressants, such as benzodiazepines and neuroleptics, may be used as adjunctive supplements, or sometimes as substitutes for antidepressants in some situations (e.g., a patient with an extremely poor prognosis who cannot wait for weeks), since antidepressants need to be taken daily, not intermittently, and require 4 to 6 weeks to achieve full effect. For any patients who have poor tolerability of antidepressants, benzodiazepines or antipsychotics, clinicians may use psychostimulants, ketamine, and cannabis because of their ultraquick action and their effectiveness for symptoms other than depression (e.g., psychostimulants for fatigue and sleepiness due to opioids; ketamine for pain; and cannabis for nausea and appetite loss).

Table 4.2 Types of Antidepressants and Their Characteristics

Drug Type	Actions	Therapeutics	Side Effects, Contraindications	Agents
Selective Serotonin Reuptake Inhibitors (SSRIs)	Blocks reuptake of serotonin (5HT) at serotonin transporter	Common initial treatment of depression. Generally mild adverse effects. Also effective for anxiety disorders	Nausea/emesis and sexual dysfunction are common. May lead to weigh gain, agitation, platelet dysfunction, insomnia or sedation.	Citalopram, Escitalopram, Fluoxetine, Fluvoxamine, Paroxetine, Sertraline
Serotonin Norepinephrine Reuptake Inhibitors (SNRIs)	Blocks reuptake of 5HT and norepinephrine (NE) at 5HT and NE transporters	Generally mild adverse effects. Also effective for neuropathic pain	High blood pressure (venlafaxine is contraindicated)	Desvenlafaxine, Venlafaxine, Duloxetine
Mirtazapine	Agonist at alpha-2 adrenergic & 5HT-2a, 2c, -3 auto receptors to facilitate release of NE & 5HT, Blocks Histamine (H1) receptors	Useful for patients with anorexia and/or insomnia	May cause weight gain, sedation, autonomic effects	Mirtazapine
Bupropion	Blocks uptake of dopamine (DA) & NE	Useful as an adjunct to SSRI. Helps with smoking cessation.	Lowered seizure threshold at higher doses (therefore, limited in palliative care)	Bupropion
Tricyclic antidepressants (TCAs)	Blocks reuptake of 5HT & NE	Secondary option for otherwise resistant depression. Limited use today, except as a coanalgesic.	Anticholinergic effects (constipation, urinary retention, confusion), arrythmia & weight gain. (contraindicated for glaucoma, past myocardial infarction & diabetes)	Amitriptyline, Clomipramine, Desipramine, Dothiepin, Doxepin, Imipramine, Nortriptyline, Protriptyline, Trimipramine
Monoamine oxidase inhibitors (MAO-Is)	Prolonged anti-MAO-A/B actions	Third-line treatment for resistant depression; not used in palliative care	Autonomic & sexual effects, Anticholinergic effects	Phenelzine, Tranylcypromine

Antidepressants

- Choice of an agent: There are a few categories ("class") of antidepressants. No single antidepressant is universally accepted as more effective than another, despite some variation in their effectiveness and acceptability.

🔍 Key Point

Initial choice of an agent should be based on adverse effects, interactions with other medications, dosing schedule, and history of effective response.

Usually, selective serotonin reuptake inhibitors (SSRIs), serotonin norepinephrine reuptake inhibitors (SNRIs), or mirtazapine are used as the first-choice drug. Treatment adherence and treatment response should be monitored twice a month, or even more (e.g., weekly) in severely depressed or suicidal patients.

- Dosage and treatment plan: Start at a low dose and titrate gradually (especially for elderly, sick, or vulnerable patients), usually at a pace of 1 to 2 weeks (see Table 4.3). SSRIs and SNRIs frequently cause nausea/emesis at the beginning of administration unless taken with food. Clinicians should inform patients that nausea/emesis may occur as an adverse effect but usually disappears within a few days. The medications should be continued for at least 6 months after reaching recovery to prevent relapse of depression.

Treatment failure should not be declared before a minimum of 4 to 6 weeks of treatment once the maximum dose is administered. The commonest reason for poor response is inadequate titration of the dosage upward, especially for patients who are rapid metabolizers.

Rotating medications (e.g., change from SSRI to SNRI) or supplementing with adjunctive medications may be indicated if there has been no response by 8 to 12 weeks at maximal dose. Typical augmentation strategies include lithium, lamotrigine, buspirone, psychostimulants, and low-dose neuroleptics (e.g., quetiapine). While the use of mood stabilizers is uncommon because of the short prognosis of patients in palliative care, use of low dose neuroleptics and psychostimulants is common.

Discontinuation syndrome can occur within days after rapid discontinuation of short-acting agents. SSRIs and SNRIs may induce dizziness, nausea, fatigue, muscle aches, chills, anxiety, and irritability. TCAs may induce agitation, sleep disturbance, flu-like symptoms, and cardiac arrythmia. Readministration of the drug alleviates those symptoms. Many antidepressants are metabolized by CYP 450; thus, clinicians should be watchful for potential interactions with other medications in use.

SSRIs/SNRIs

SSRIs are the most frequently prescribed antidepressants. Postcibal administration (e.g., taken after breakfast) reduces the risk of nausea. Antiemetic drugs (e.g., mosapride, metoclopramide) can be prescribed for these side effects. Other common adverse effects include sleep disturbance (either insomnia or hypersomnia) and sexual dysfunction, although the latter is less relevant in palliative care. Since serotonin associates with platelet aggregation, administration of SSRIs can increase the risk of bleeding (bleeding

Table 4.3 Initial and Regular Dose of Medications

Medication	Initial Dose (mg/day)	Dosing Range (mg/day)	Key Drug Interactions
SSRIs			**Caution with NSAIDS (risk of bleeding) and diuretics (SIADH)**
Citalopram	10–20	20–60	
Escitalopram	5–10	10–20	
Fluoxetine	10–20	20–80	
Fluvoxamine	25–50	50–300	
Paroxetine	10–20	20–60 (CR: 2.5–62.5)	CYP 2D6 inhibition (may affect Tamoxifen metabolism)
Sertraline	25–50	50–200	
SNRIs			**Caution with ciprofloxacin, ketoconazole**
Desvenlafaxine	50	50–150	
Duloxetine	30	30–120	
Venlafaxine	75	25–300	
Other antidepressants			
Bupropion	25–50	150–450	May lower seizure threshold
Buspirone	15	15–60	
Mirtazapine	15	15–45	
Psychostimulants			**Caution with antihypertensive medications, clonidine, anticoagulants, steroids, anticonvulsants**
Methylphenidate	5–10	20	
Modafinil	50–100	100–200	

diatheses), especially for the patients who are already taking NSAIDs or other antiplatelet medications. Syndrome of inappropriate antidiuretic hormone secretion (SIADH) [low sodium and low serum osmolality] can be caused by SSRIs and SNRIs (and tricyclics).

In a small group of individuals, SSRIs and SNRIs may cause irritability, agitation, or dysphoria at the beginning of administration ("activation syndrome"). This can be alleviated by decreasing the dose, switching medicine, or concurrently using benzodiazepines. Abrupt stopping of an SSRI or SNRI can present with severe dizziness, fatigue, and dysphoria, arising from readaptation of receptors ("withdrawal syndrome"), thus they should be tapered rather than be stopped abruptly. Readministration of the drug alleviates those symptoms.

Mirtazapine
In contrast to SSRIs/SNRIs, mirtazapine usually does not cause nausea or emesis. Rather, it increases appetite and is favored by patients who suffer from appetite loss not only due to depression but also due to cancer progression and cancer treatment. Sleepiness is another common adverse effect that can be either harmful or helpful for patients depending on their situation (i.e. somnolence can decrease patients' function but can be helpful for those who suffer from insomnia).

Bupropion
Bupropion is often used as an adjunct to serotonin-reuptake inhibitors; however, it is evolving into the favored drug for inflammatory depressions. It also helps with smoking cessation.

Tricyclics
Tricyclic antidepressants (TCAs) are older-generation antidepressants that have more frequent adverse effects and lower tolerability. Since their effectiveness is not significantly different from those of newer generation antidepressants (e.g., SSRIs/SNRIs, mirtazapine, bupropion), TCAs are seldom used as a first-line antidepressant. Some TCAs may be used because of their coanalgesic effects. Their anticholinergic effects may cause constipation and may need to be avoided by patients at a risk of bowel obstruction, and they may cause urinary retention.

Monoamine Oxidase Inhibitors
Monoamine oxidase inhibitors (MAO-Is) have many harmful adverse effects (autonomic effects and dietary restrictions [avoid tyramine]) and are thus considered a third-line treatment for resistant depression. They are seldom used in palliative care settings.

Benzodiazepines
Benzodiazepines are the most commonly used anxiolytics, which may be used as an adjunct to antidepressants to alleviate distress, anxiety, and/or agitation. Their quick effect is considered favorable by patients and clinicians, although their effectiveness for depression in the long term (> four weeks) has not been proven. Benzodiazepines are also frequently used as hypnotics. The same cautions apply as those for anxiolytics.

Common adverse effects of benzodiazepines are sleepiness, fatigue, and decreased concentration, which can impair daily functioning. They may also cause dizziness and muscle weakness (due to its muscle-relaxant effect), which can create a risk of falls. Benzodiazepines may induce delirium in vulnerable patients, such as older patients or those with advanced illness. All benzodiazepines are metabolized in the liver and have active metabolites, except for lorazepam, which is metabolized through glucuronidation without active metabolites; therefore, lorazepam is relatively safely used for patients with liver dysfunction.

Buspirone

Buspirone is another anxiolytic whose adverse effects are milder than benzodiazepines. Although its effectiveness as a sole agent in treating depression is limited, its adjunctive use with SSRIs can be helpful.

Neuroleptics

Neuroleptics (can be termed antipsychotics, although this is a stigmatized word that is unhelpful for the medically ill) are used either as an augmentation therapy for depression or as an alternative for anxiolytics, especially for patients with severe symptoms that cannot be alleviated by benzodiazepines or for patients at risk of dependence using benzodiazepines. Some neuroleptics (e.g., quetiapine, aripiprazole) themselves have antidepressant effects. Their potential adverse effects include extrapyramidal symptoms (Parkinsonian syndrome) and weight gain, the latter being helpful in palliative care.

Psychostimulants

Psychostimulants, such as methylphenidate and modafinil, are used to counter fatigue/sedation from opioids and help depression near the end of life. They can be used alone if rapid onset is needed, or in combination with traditional antidepressants to get an initial response faster or as an adjunct.

Ketamine

Ketamine has been increasingly recognized as a reasonable option for depressed patients who are resistant to antidepressants or who need immediate resolution of depression (such as patients who are seriously suicidal). Also, it may be used in palliative care as an infusion to relieve a pain crisis. The effects of ketamine on both pain and depression are considered favorable in palliative care settings. Ketamine is usually administered intravenously, but may be administered subcutaneously or intranasally in some situations.

Cannabis

Cannabis may be prescribed in some jurisdictions, although so far there is no supportive evidence base to prescribe cannabis for the treatment of depression.

Psilocybin

Studies have begun to trial the use of psilocybin in conjunction with intensive psychotherapy in the setting of advanced cancer.

Electroconvulsive Therapy

Electroconvulsive therapy (ECT) is a maneuver to induce controlled seizure using electrical stimulation in the brain while the patient is under anesthesia. It is the most established somatic therapy as a treatment of choice for patients with depression refractory to pharmacotherapy, patients with psychotic depression, patients who are acutely suicidal, and vulnerable patients (e.g., the elderly, Parkinson's) who cannot tolerate standard pharmacotherapy. There are no absolute contraindications, however caution may be needed for those with cardiovascular disease (because of transient increase in heart rate and blood pressure from ECT) and brain tumors/increased intracranial pressure (risk of prolonged seizures). The common adverse effects of ECT include transient headache and muscle ache, dental fractures and oral trauma, arrhythmias, transient cognitive dysfunction (acute confusion and/or short-term amnesia). Although the use of ECT in cancer has not been well-studied, several case studies suggest its safety and effectiveness. It has occasional merit in palliative care when the prognosis is measured in months and cerebral metastases have been excluded.

Other Neuromodulation Therapies

Other neuromodulation therapies for depression include transcranial magnetic stimulation (TMS) and transcranial direct current stimulation (tDCS). Although clinical evidence of these therapies in palliative care settings has been scarce, they may be applicable in some situations and when available.

TMS stimulates the prefrontal cortex through an induced magnetic field. The treatment is usually given approximately 5 days a week for 4 to 6 weeks; hence its utility in palliative care is very limited. The possible adverse effects of TMS include seizure, scalp pain from stimulation of muscles and nerves, headache, and light-headedness. Intracranial metal implants, history of stroke, pregnancy, and poorly controlled migraines are among its contraindications.

Complementary and Integrative Therapies

Systematic reviews show that meditation, yoga, relaxation with imagery, massage, and music therapy may be helpful for patients with depressive disorders with cancer, although the methodologic quality of the referenced studies is generally low.

Mindfulness-based interventions, especially mindfulness-based stress reduction (MBSR) and mindfulness-based cognitive therapy (MBCT), have a strong evidence-base to reduce depression and other stress-related symptoms in patients with cancer.

Professional Issues and Service Implementation

Recording and Communicating

As described earlier, "depression" is a term used by many health professionals for the usual sadness resulting from a medical diagnosis. When a clinician uses the term "depression," we must clarify what the term refers to clinically. Some patients may benefit from receiving an audio recording of the consultation as a communication aid.

Severe Depression's Impact on Mental Capacity

Patients with severe depression are at elevated risk of suicide. If a patient is suspected to be at urgent risk of suicide, intensive psychiatric care, including one-to-one inpatient companionship on the oncology ward for safety, or admission to a psychiatric ward is indicated, depending on the nursing and medical care needed. In many countries, involuntary admission is permitted for patients who are at immediate risk of suicide, but most psychiatric wards are not set up to manage the terminally ill. The solution is to have a very clear protocol on the oncology/palliative care ward in terms of management of suicide risk, with a psychiatric consultation occurring in this palliative care setting. Clinicians are responsible for informing the caregivers of the risk, as well as referring such patients to an appropriate mental healthcare specialist. Severe depression may interfere with a patient's appreciation of the prognosis and limit decision-making capacity.

Common Ethical Dilemmas

Depression is a large contributor to the wish for hastened death (e.g., through suicide, physician-assisted suicide, euthanasia, or rejection of proper treatment). Clinicians should be cautious about the presence of depression and its influence on patients with such requests. It is not always easy to discriminate clinical depression from a patient's natural response to tough physical conditions. The rule of thumb is to prioritize the diagnosis of depression in order not to miss the chance of recovery that can be attained (see also Chapter 6 for more on managing desire for hastened death).

Policies

Because of the high prevalence and remarkable impact of depression on patients' quality of life, some societies mandate routine screening of psychological distress (mainly targeting depression) in oncology practice. For example, the American College of Surgeons Commission on Cancer mandated implementation of a systematic protocol for distress screening and referral as a condition for cancer center accreditation starting in 2015. In Japan, the provision of distress screening is required in order to be certified as a registered cancer center.

Teams and Supervision

Regardless of whether the patient is diagnosed as depressed, any bio- or psychosocial problems and concerns should be addressed through an interdisciplinary approach, which involves collaboration with and referral to appropriate disciplines when necessary. Detection and management of depression may be best done by collaboration between frontline medical providers (e.g., primary care physicians or oncologists) and a trained "care manager" (e.g., trained nurses) who work under the supervision of consultant psychiatrists. A typical program of this "collaborative care model" starts with the administration of a self-report screening questionnaire for depression to all the patients in a clinic. If a patient reports high emotional distress, he or she receives a face-to-face or telephone diagnostic interview for depression by trained staff. If the patient is diagnosed with depression, he or she is provided with psychoeducation for depression and brief psychotherapy (usually brief CBT such as problem-solving therapy), in addition to practical advice on managing life with cancer and psychological distress. When clinically relevant, a report is generated for the patient's primary care provider. Also, guidance about the use of psychotropics is provided by the care managers under the supervision of psychiatrists.

References

1. Caruso R, Nanni MG, Riba M, et al. Depressive spectrum disorders in cancer: Prevalence, risk factors and screening for depression: A critical review. Acta Oncol 2017;56(2):146–155.

2. Mitchell AJ, Chan M, Bhatti H, et al. Prevalence of depression, anxiety, and adjustment disorder in oncological, haematological, and palliative-care settings: A meta-analysis of 94 interview-based studies. Lancet Oncol. 2011;12(2):160–174.

3. Walker J, Holm Hansen C, Martin P, et al. Prevalence of depression in adults with cancer: A systematic review. Ann Oncol. 2013;24:895–900.

4. Janberidze E, Hjermstad MJ, Haugen DF, EURO IMPACT, et al. How are patient populations characterized in studies investigating depression in advanced cancer? Results from a systematic literature review. J Pain Symptom Manage. 2014;48:678–698.

5. National Institute for Health and Care Excellence (NICE): Depression in adults with a chronic physical health problem: Recognition and management (CG91). NICE 2009. Clinical guideline published: October 28, 2009. nice.org.uk/guidance/cg91..

6. Fujisawa D, Inoguchi H, Shimoda H, et al. Impact of depression on health utility value in cancer patients. Psycho-Oncology.. 2015;25(5):491–495. https://onlinelibrary.wiley.com/doi/10.1002/pon.3945

7. Pirl WF, Greer JA, Traeger L, et al. Depression and survival in metastatic non–small-cell lung cancer: Effects of early palliative care. J Clin Oncol. 2012;30(12):1310–1315.

8. Warnke I, Nordt C, Kawohl W, Moock J, Rössler W. Age- and gender-specific mortality risk profiles for depressive outpatients with major chronic medical diseases. J Affect Disord. 2016;193:295–304. https://doi.org/10.1016/j.jad.2016.01.006.

9. Mausbach BT, Schwab RB, Irwin SA. Depression as a predictor of adherence to adjuvant endocrine therapy (AET) in women with breast cancer: A systematic review and meta-analysis. Breast Cancer Res Treat. 2015;152(2):239–246. https://doi.org/10.1007/s10549-015-3471-7.

10. Fujisawa D, Temel JS, Traeger L, Greer JA, Lennes IT, Mimura M, Pirl WF. Psychological factors at early stage of treatment as predictors of receiving chemotherapy at the end of life. Psycho-Oncology. 2015;24(12):1731–1737.

11. Oliveira Miranda D, Soares de Lima TA, Ribeiro Azevedo L, Feres O, Ribeiro da Rocha JJ, Pereira-da-Silva G. Proinflammatory cytokines correlate with depression and anxiety in colorectal cancer patients. Biomed Res Int. 2014;739650. https://doi.org/10.1155/2014/739650.

12. Sullivan M, Youngner S. Depression, competence, and the right to refuse lifesaving medical treatment. Am J Psychiatry. 1994;151:971–978.

13. Walker J, Waters RA, Murray G, et al. Better off dead: Suicidal thoughts in cancer patients. J Clin Oncol. 2008;26:4725–4730.

14. Felger JC, Lotrich FE. Inflammatory cytokines in depression: Neurobiological mechanisms and therapeutic implications. Neuroscience 2013;246:199–229.

15. Raison CL, Miller AH. Depression in cancer: New developments regarding diagnosis and treatment. Biol Psychiatry. 2003;54(3):283–294.

16. National Comprehensive Cancer Network. NCCN Clinical Practice Guidelines in Oncology: Distress Management, Version 2, 2022. https://www.nccn.org/guidelines/guidelines-detail?category=3&id=1431

17. Ostuzzi G, Matcham F, Dauchy S, Barbui C, Hotopf M. Antidepressants for the treatment of depression in people with cancer. Cochrane Database Syst Rev. 2018;4(4):CD011006.

18. Li M, Kennedy EB, Byrne N, et al. Systematic review and meta-analysis of collaborative care interventions for depression in patients with cancer. Psychooncology. 2017;26(5):573–587.

19. Okuyama T, Akechi T, Mackenzie L, Furukawa TA. Psychotherapy for depression among advanced, incurable cancer patients: A systematic review and meta-analysis. Cancer Treat Rev. 2017;56:16–27.

20. Rodin G, An E, Shnall J, Malfitano C. Psychological interventions for patients with advanced disease: Implications for oncology and palliative care. J Clin Oncol. 2020;38(9):885–904.

21. Andrew BN, Guan NC, Jaafar NRN. The use of methylphenidate for physical and psychological symptoms in cancer patients: A review. Curr Drug Targets. 2018;19(8):877–887.

22. Dean RL, Hurducas C, Hawton K, et al. Ketamine and other glutamate receptor modulators for depression in adults with unipolar major depressive disorder. Cochrane Database Syst Rev. 2021;9(9):CD011612.

23. Cillessen L, Johannsen M, Speckens AEM, Zachariae R. Mindfulness-based interventions for psychological and physical health outcomes in cancer patients and survivors: A systematic review and meta-analysis of randomized controlled trials. Psycho-Oncology. 2019;28(12):2257–2269.

24. Agboola SO, Ju W, Elfiky A, Kvedar JC, Jethwani K. The effect of technology-based interventions on pain, depression, and quality of life in patients with cancer: A systematic review of randomized controlled trials. J Med Internet Res. 2015;17(3):e65.

25. Willems RA, Bolman CAW, Lechner L, et al. Online interventions aimed at reducing psychological distress in cancer patients: Evidence update and suggestions for future directions. Curr Opin Support Palliat Care. 2020;14(1):27–39.

26. Caruso R, Nanni M, Riba MB, Sabato S, Grassi L. Depressive spectrum disorders in cancer: Diagnostic issues and intervention. A critical review. Curr Psychiatry Rep. 2017;19(6):33.

27. Lie HC, Hjermstad MJ, Fayers P, Finset A, Kaasa S, Loge JH. European Palliative Care Research Collaborative (EPCRC). Depression in advanced cancer-assessment challenges and associations with disease load. J Affect Disord. 2015;173:176–184.

28. Wakefield CE, Butow PN, Aaronson NA, et al. Patient-reported depression measures in cancer: A meta-review. Lancet Psychiatry. 2015;2(7):635–647.

Further Reading

Andersen BL, DeRubeis RJ, Berman BS, et al., for the American Society of Clinical Oncology. Screening, assessment, and care of anxiety and depressive symptoms in adults with cancer: An American Society of Clinical Oncology guideline adaptation. J Clin Oncol. 2014;32(15):1605–16019. Guidelines proposed by ASCO for the treatment of depression in cancer care.

Howell D, Keller-Olaman S, Oliver T, et al. A pan-Canadian practice guideline: Screening, assessment and care of psychosocial distress (depression, anxiety) in adults with cancer. Canadian Partnership Against Cancer (Cancer Journey Action Group) and the Canadian Association of Psychosocial Oncology, 2010. Canadian guidelines proposed by CAPO and CJAG.

National Comprehensive Cancer Network. NCCN Clinical Practice Guidelines (NCCN Guidelines) Distress Management version 2. 2021. NCCN Distress Screening guideline.

Watson M, Kissane DW, Editors. Management of Clinical Depression and Anxiety. New York: Oxford University Press; 2017. A recent IPOS-supported set of guidelines for the management of anxiety and depression in general cancer care.

Watson M, Kissane DW, Editors. Handbook of Psychotherapy in Cancer Care. Wiley; 2011. Comprehensive outline of the models of psychotherapy delivered in cancer care.

Breitbart W, et al. Psycho-Oncology, 4th ed. New York: Oxford University Press; 2021. Comprehensive textbook about psycho-oncology as a discipline.

Chapter 5

Delirium and Cognitive Impairment

Yesne Alici, Soenke Boettger, and William S. Breitbart

Learning Objectives

After reading this chapter, the clinician will be able to:

1. Understand the epidemiology, common clinical features, differential diagnosis, and assessment of delirium in cancer patients in palliative care settings
2. Differentiate acute from chronic cognitive changes and understand their clinical implications
3. Differentiate reversible delirium from terminal delirium at the end of life
4. Demonstrate key management principles in responding to delirium and other cognitive disorders in the palliative care setting
5. Describe ethical, cultural, legal, and professional issues that may arise in the clinical care of patients with delirium and other cognitive disorders in the palliative care setting

Background Evidence

Delirium is a common and often serious neuropsychiatric complication in the management of terminally ill patients, characterized by abrupt onset of disturbances in awareness, attention, cognition, and perception that fluctuates over the course of the day.[1] Delirium is associated with increased morbidity and mortality and increased length of hospital stay, causing distress in patients, family members, and staff.[2] Delirium is a sign of significant physiologic disturbance, usually involving multiple medical etiologies, such as infection, organ failure, and medication adverse effects. Delirium can interfere with the recognition and control of other physical symptoms, such as pain. Unfortunately, delirium is often underrecognized or misdiagnosed, inappropriately treated, or left untreated in the medical setting. Clinicians working in palliative care settings must be able to diagnose delirium accurately, undertake appropriate assessment of etiologies, and understand the benefits and risks of pharmacologic and nonpharmacologic interventions currently available.

Delirium is the most prevalent neuropsychiatric disorder in palliative care settings.[3-5] The reported prevalence and incidence of delirium varies widely in the medical literature. This is due to the diverse and complex nature of delirium and the heterogeneity of sample populations. The prevalence of delirium at admission to general medical and geriatric wards ranges from 18% to 35%, and the incidence of delirium during such hospitalization ranges from 29% to 64%.[2] Old age is a well-known risk factor for the development of delirium, as is dementia or other cognitive impairment, functional impairment, visual impairment, and a history of alcohol use disorders. Postoperative patients, cancer patients, and acquired immunodeficiency syndrome (AIDS) patients are also at greater risk for delirium. Delirium occurs in up to 51% of postoperative patients. Approximately 25%–40% of medically hospitalized cancer patients develop delirium, as do about 85% of terminally ill cancer patients.[6,7] Advanced or severe illness involving multiorgan systems increases the risk of developing delirium. The highest prevalence and incidence of delirium is reported in hospice settings with terminally ill patients. Prospective studies conducted in inpatient palliative care units have found an occurrence rate of delirium ranging from 13% to 42% on admission, and incident delirium developing during this admission in 26% to 62%.[6]

As reflected by its diverse phenomenology, delirium is a dysfunction of multiple regions of the brain, a global cerebral dysfunction characterized by concurrent disturbances of levels of alertness, awareness, attention, perception, cognition, psychomotor behavior, mood, and sleep-wake cycle. Fluctuations of these symptoms, as well as the abrupt onset of such disturbances are critical features of delirium. Delirium is conceptualized as a reversible process as opposed to dementia. Reversibility is often possible even in severely ill patients; however, irreversible or persistent delirium has been described in the last days of life as terminal delirium. Studies within the last decade have also shown long-term cognitive impairment as a result of prolonged and severe delirium episodes.

Various hypotheses have been put forth to explain the pathophysiology of delirium, including neuronal aging, neuroinflammation, oxidative stress, neuroendocrine disturbance, circadian rhythm dysregulation, and neurotransmitter hypotheses; none of them are mutually exclusive. Variable contribution of these hypotheses may lead to the development of cognitive and behavioral dysfunctions characteristics of delirium.[8]

Presenting Problems

The clinical features of delirium include a variety of neuropsychiatric symptoms (see Box 5.1). The main features of delirium include prodromal symptoms (e.g., restlessness, anxiety, sleep disturbances, and irritability), rapidly fluctuating course, abrupt onset of symptoms representing a change from baseline over hours to days, reduced attention (e.g., distractibility), altered awareness of surroundings, altered level of alertness (e.g., hypoalert), increased or decreased psychomotor activity, disturbance of sleep-wake cycle, affective symptoms (e.g., emotional lability, depressed mood, anger,

---

Box 5.1 Clinical Features of Delirium

Disturbance in level of alertness

Attention impairment

Rapidly fluctuating course and abrupt onset of symptoms

Increased or decreased psychomotor activity

Disturbance of sleep-wake cycle

Mood symptoms and lability

Perceptual disturbances

Disorganized thinking

Incoherent speech

Disorientation and memory impairment

Other cognitive impairments (e.g., word-finding difficulty, visuospatial dysfunction)

Neurological findings: Asterixis, frontal release signs

---

or euphoria), perceptual disturbances (e.g., misperceptions, illusions, and hallucinations), delusions, disorganized thinking and incoherent speech, disorientation, and memory impairment. Language disturbance may be evident as dysnomia, dysgraphia, or more commonly word-finding difficulties. Speech may be rambling, pressured, and incoherent. Neurologic abnormalities may include asterixis, or frontal release signs.

Phenomenology studies have shown cognitive impairment to be common with disorientation occurring in 78%–100%, attention deficits in 62%–100%, memory deficits in 62%–90%, and diffuse cognitive deficits in 77%; disturbance of consciousness was recorded in 65%–100% of patients with delirium; disorganized thinking was found in 95%, language abnormalities in 47%–93%, and sleep-wake cycle disturbances in 49%–96%.

It is important to note that the degree of cognitive impairment and the domains affected may vary; therefore, the testing of a single domain of cognition, such as orientation, may lead to underrecognition of delirium. The cognitive assessment of patients at risk for delirium should include testing of multiple domains, at the very least, orientation, attention, recall, and language functioning.

According to the Diagnostic and Statistical Manual of Mental Disorders, fifth edition (DSM-5), the essential features of delirium are:

- disrupted attention (e.g., difficulty directing, focusing, sustaining, or shifting attention) and awareness (i.e., reduced orientation to the environment);
- a change from baseline that develops over hours to days and fluctuates within a day;
- additional cognitive problems (e.g., in memory, orientation, language, visuospatial ability, or perception);
- the condition is not better explained by another neurocognitive disorder and is not associated with a state of severely reduced arousal, such as coma;

- history, physical examination, or laboratory findings suggest the patient's mental state is a direct physiological result of another medical condition, substance intoxication or withdrawal, exposure to a toxin, or multiple etiological factors.

The abrupt onset and fluctuation of the signs and symptoms are integral parts of the diagnostic criteria. DSM-5, like the previous edition of the manual, does not place diagnostic emphasis on disturbance of the sleep-wake cycle or disturbances in psychomotor activity.

Clinically, the diagnostic gold standard for delirium is the clinician's assessment utilizing the DSM-5 criteria. Several delirium screening and evaluation tools have been developed to maximize diagnostic precision for clinical and research purposes, and to assess delirium severity.

✔ Tools

Examples of delirium assessment tools used in cancer patients and in palliative care settings include:

- Memorial Delirium Assessment Scale (MDAS),
- 4 A's Test for Delirium (4AT),
- Confusion Assessment Method (CAM), and
- Mini-Mental State Exam (MMSE).

Each of these scales has good reliability and validity. Use of the CAM has also been extended to mechanically ventilated patients in intensive care units (ICUs) with the creation of the CAM-ICU.

Depending on the underlying etiologies, there may be additional presenting signs or symptoms that may help the clinician in their diagnostic inquiry.

🔍 Key Point

Serotonin syndrome, a frequently underrecognized condition that develops with use of multiple serotonergic agents, such as serotonergic antidepressants, opioids, and tramadol, has a distinct presentation. Mild symptoms include nervousness, insomnia, nausea, diarrhea, tremor, and dilated pupils, which can then progress to moderate symptoms such as hyperreflexia, diaphoresis, agitation, restlessness, clonus, and ocular clonus.

Patients with severe symptoms should be referred to the hospital immediately. The nervousness, insomnia, agitation, restlessness described above are a part of the delirium due to serotonin syndrome. In the absence of a keen review of medications and a neurological examination, the etiology is likely to be missed for this reversible condition in palliative care settings. Catatonic features may point to a neuroleptic malignant syndrome or autoimmune encephalopathy, the latter of which should be in the differential in the era of immunotherapies.

Based on the psychomotor behavior, three subtypes of delirium are described. The three subtypes include:

- hyperactive (or agitated, or hyperalert) subtype;
- hypoactive (or lethargic, hypoalert, or hypoaroused) subtype; and
- mixed subtype (alternating features of hypo- and hyperactive delirium).

The **hypoactive subtype** is characterized by psychomotor retardation, lethargy, sedation, and reduced awareness of surroundings. Hypoactive delirium is often mistaken for depression and is difficult to differentiate from sedation due to opioids, or obtundation in the last days of life.

The **hyperactive subtype** is commonly characterized by restlessness, agitation, hypervigilance, hallucinations, and delusions. Hyperactive delirium is more easily recognized by clinicians due to increased psychomotor activity and is more likely to be referred to psychiatrists compared to patients with other subtypes of delirium.

In the palliative care setting, hypoactive delirium is most common. It is important to note that patients with hypoactive delirium may also experience hallucinations and delusions, requiring treatment of these distressing symptoms. Both hypoactive and hyperactive subtypes of delirium have been shown to cause distress in patients, family members, clinicians, and staff.[9] Patients with hypoactive delirium (i.e., with few outward manifestations of discomfort or distress) have been found to be just as distressed as patients with hyperactive delirium.[9,10]

Case Study

Anthony is a 57-year-old man with recently diagnosed metastatic pancreatic cancer, currently on gemcitabine, who presents to the emergency room with altered mental status. He is noted to be disoriented, inattentive, with word finding difficulty. He becomes irritable on exam, refusing to cooperate with questions to assess his cognition. He is guarded with notable paranoia throughout the assessment. His wife at the bedside reports, "This is not him! He is the kindest person you can imagine. What has cancer done to my husband?" Bloodwork reveals severe dehydration. His imaging is of concern for progression of disease. Assessment also reveals that Anthony was started on morphine around the clock for severe back pain two days prior. Anthony is admitted for further assessment and work up. He is started on intravenous fluids. Morphine is switched over to fentanyl due to concern for its contribution to altered mental status. On exam the next morning, he remains mildly disoriented, with notable improvements in attention and paranoia. Anthony and his wife are provided information on delirium, the multifactorial nature of it, and the reversibility with treatment of the underlying etiologies. A palliative care consultation is requested for a goals of care discussion.

Investigations for Key Differential Diagnoses

In the palliative care setting, delirium can result either from the direct effects of the primary illness on the central nervous system (CNS), secondary illnesses arising independently, or from the indirect CNS effects of diseases or treatments (e.g., medications, electrolyte imbalance, dehydration, major organ failure, infection, vascular complications, or autoimmune/paraneoplastic encephalitis).[7] Box 5.2 provides a summary of potentially reversible contributors to delirium. There is evidence suggesting that the

---

Box 5.2 Potentially Reversible Factors Contributing to Delirium

Medication/substance use (e.g., steroids, benzodiazepines, anticholinergic medications)

Medication/substance withdrawal (e.g., alcohol withdrawal)

Medication/substance interaction (e.g., use of multiple serotonergic agents leading to serotonin syndrome)

Electrolyte and metabolic disturbances

Nutritional deficiency (e.g., thiamine deficiency)

Dehydration

Hypoxia

Infections

Bowel/bladder obstruction/retention

Pain

---

subtypes of delirium may be related to different causes. Hypoactive delirium has generally been found to occur due to hypoxia, metabolic disturbances, and hepatic encephalopathies. Hyperactive delirium is correlated with alcohol and drug withdrawal, drug intoxication, or medication adverse effects.

The diagnostic workup of delirium should include an assessment for these potentially reversible causes. The clinician should obtain a detailed history from family, caregivers, and staff of the patient's baseline mental status, and determine whether an abrupt change in mental status or fluctuating mental status is present. It is important to inquire about alcohol or other substance use disorders in hospitalized patients to be able to recognize and treat alcohol or other substance-induced withdrawal delirium appropriately. A full physical examination should assess for evidence of sepsis, dehydration, or major organ failure (renal, hepatic, pulmonary). Medications that could contribute to delirium should be reviewed and possible medication interactions should be carefully considered. Opioid analgesics, benzodiazepines, and anticholinergic drugs are common causes of delirium, particularly in the elderly and the terminally ill. The challenge of assessing the relative contribution of medications to an episode of delirium is often compounded by the presence of many other potential contributors to cognitive changes, such as infection, metabolic disturbance, dehydration, pain, or medication withdrawal.

Assessment and management of pain plays a significant role in management of patients in palliative care settings. Inadequate pain control can trigger delirium, as well as inappropriate pain medication use. The successful treatment of pain is highly dependent on proper assessment. The assessment of pain intensity becomes very difficult in patients with delirium. Delirium can interfere dramatically with the recognition and control of pain, and other physical and psychological symptoms in advanced cancer patients, particularly in the terminally ill. Patients with severe pain are particularly at risk of delirium due to their high opioid requirements. Due to reversal of sleep-wake cycle, patients with delirium use a significantly greater number of "break-through" doses of opioids at night compared to patients without delirium. In turn, agitation may be misinterpreted as uncontrolled pain, resulting in inappropriate escalation of opioids, potentially exacerbating delirium. Accurate pain reporting depends on the ability to perceive the pain normally and to communicate the experience appropriately. Delirium may impair the ability to both perceive and report pain accurately. Patients' ability to manage their own pain through patient-controlled analgesia should be considered carefully where applicable. Efforts have been made to improve assessment of pain in nonverbal palliative care patients and some pain management strategies show promise of reducing pain without increasing the risk of delirium.

🔍 Key Point

Reducing the dose of opioids or switching to another opioid has been demonstrated to reverse delirium due to opioids.

Laboratory Investigations

A screen of laboratory parameters (see Table 5.1) will allow assessment of the possible role of metabolic abnormalities, such as hypercalcemia or thiamine deficiency, and other problems, such as hypoxia or disseminated intravascular coagulation (DIC). In some instances, an EEG (e.g., to rule out seizures), brain imaging studies (e.g., to rule out brain metastases, intracranial bleeding, or ischemia), D-dimer (to rule out DIC) or CT angiogram of chest to rule out pulmonary embolism, and lumbar puncture (e.g., to rule

Table 5.1 Delirium Workup and Potential Etiologies

Delirium Workup*	Reasons for Tests—Potential Etiologies
Basic metabolic panel	Electrolyte disturbances, acute renal insufficiency, dehydration
Liver function tests, ammonia levels	Hepatic insufficiency, hepatic encephalopathy
Complete blood count	Infections, anemia, hypercoagulability, disseminated intravascular coagulation
Arterial blood gas	Hypoxia, hypercarbia
Urinalysis and culture	Urinary tract infection, renal insufficiency
Blood cultures	Sepsis
Thiamine levels	Nonalcoholic Wernicke's encephalopathy
Electrocardiogram	Acute myocardial infarct, sinus tachycardia
Chest X Ray or CT	Pneumonia, pulmonary embolism
Thyroid function tests	Hyper- or hypothyroidism
CT, MRI Brain	Intracranial edema, intracranial bleed or infarcts, new-onset brain metastases
EEG	Seizures
Lumbar puncture, autoimmune panel	Leptomeningeal disease, intracranial infections, autoimmune encephalitis

*Specific tests should be guided by history, physical examination, and previous results. Diagnostic workup must be consistent with the goals of care, and minimally invasive in the terminally ill. Treatments that are effective and/or minimally burdensome or distressing can be considered if congruent with goals of care.

out leptomeningeal carcinomatosis, subarachnoid hemorrhage, or meningitis) may be appropriate.

In light of the several studies on reversibility of delirium, the prognosis of patients who develop delirium is defined by the interaction of the patient's baseline physiologic susceptibility to delirium (e.g., predisposing factors), the precipitating etiologies, and any response to treatment. If a patient's susceptibility or resilience is modifiable, then targeted interventions may reduce the risk of delirium upon exposure to a precipitant and enhance the capacity to respond to treatment. Conversely, if a patient is frail, then exposure to precipitants enhances the likelihood of developing delirium and may diminish the probability of a complete restoration of cognitive function.

Differential Diagnoses of Delirium

Many of the clinical features of delirium can also be associated with other psychiatric disorders, such as depression, mania, psychosis, and dementia, making diagnosis particularly challenging (see Table 5.2). Due to delirium's fluctuating course, there can be disagreement between clinicians evaluating the patient at different times of day about whether there is any abnormality at all. Assessments that differ widely between time points within the same day are suggestive of delirium.

▸ **Depressive disorders:** When delirium presents with mood symptoms such as depression, apathy, euphoria, or irritability, these symptoms are not uncommonly attributed to depression or mania, especially in patients

Table 5.2 Differential Diagnosis of Cognitive Impairment in Palliative Care Settings	
Diagnosis	**Differentiating Features**
Delirium	**Delirium**—acute onset, fluctuating course, delusions or hallucinations can be present in addition to cognitive impairment
Delirium and Dementia	**Delirium superimposed on dementia or mild cognitive impairment**—typically seen in the elderly. These patients typically have known underlying cognitive impairment that gets acutely worse in the setting of delirium due to medical etiologies or medications. History taking from caregivers is essential for diagnosis.
Dementia or Major Cognitive Disorder	**Dementia or major neurocognitive disorder**—insidious onset, collateral information, the longitudinal review of signs and symptoms help determine the diagnosis. Cognitive impairments interfere with day-to-day functioning. The etiologies vary from neurodegenerative illness (e.g., Parkinson's), to cancer treatments, or cerebrovascular disease. Commonly multifactorial in palliative care settings.
Mild Cognitive Disorder	**Mild cognitive impairment or mild neurocognitive disorder**—insidious onset, collateral information, the longitudinal review of signs and symptoms help determine the diagnosis. Cognitive impairments do not interfere with day-to-day functioning. The etiologies vary from neurodegenerative illness, to cancer treatments, or cerebrovascular disease. Commonly multifactorial in palliative care settings.

with a past psychiatric or family history of these conditions. The hypoactive subtype of delirium is commonly misdiagnosed as depression. Symptoms of major depression, including decreased psychomotor activity, insomnia, reduced ability to concentrate, depressed mood, and even suicidal ideation, can overlap with symptoms of delirium.

🔍 Key Point
In distinguishing delirium from depression, particularly in the context of advanced cancer, an evaluation of the onset and temporal sequencing of depressive and cognitive symptoms is particularly helpful.

It is important to note that the degree of cognitive impairment is much more pronounced in delirium than in depression, and delirium has a more abrupt onset. Also, in delirium the characteristic disturbance in level of alertness is present, while this is not usually a feature of depression.

- **Manic disorder:** Similarly, a manic episode may share some features with delirium, particularly the hyperactive or mixed subtypes; however, it is not common for mania to present with any disturbances in level of alertness or with the degree of cognitive deficits seen in delirium.
- **Anxiety and panic disorder:** Symptoms such as severe anxiety and autonomic hyperactivity can lead the clinician to an erroneous diagnosis of a panic attack. Review of the time course is crucial; a panic attack reaches its peak and remits within minutes, delirium fluctuates throughout the day.
- **Psychotic disorders:** Delirium causing vivid hallucinations and delusions must be distinguished from schizophrenia spectrum disorders. Delusions in delirium tend to be poorly organized and of abrupt onset, while hallucinations are predominantly visual or tactile, rather than auditory, as is typical of schizophrenia. Acute onset, fluctuating course, disturbances of cognition, and reduced awareness of surroundings, in the presence of one or more etiologic causes, are helpful in differentiating delirium from other psychiatric disorders.
- **Other cognitive disorders:** These present a diagnostic challenge more so in the palliative care setting due to the multifactorial nature of etiologies (See Table 5.2). The question comes up whether the patient has delirium, dementia, or a delirium superimposed on a preexisting dementia. Both delirium and dementia are disorders of cognition and share common clinical features, such as disorientation, memory impairment, aphasia, apraxia, agnosia, and executive dysfunction. Impairments in judgment, abstract thinking, and disturbances in thought process are seen in both disorders. Furthermore, delusions and hallucinations can be central features of certain types of dementia (e.g., Lewy body dementia). Collateral informants who can attest to the patient's baseline cognitive function are indispensable in differentiating the delirium from dementia. Abrupt onset, fluctuating course, and disturbance of arousal differentiate delirium from dementia. The temporal onset of symptoms in dementia is insidious and the course is chronically progressive. In delirium superimposed on a premorbid dementia, differential diagnosis becomes even more challenging. Signs of dementia that might otherwise be obvious tend to be obscured by the

more acute signs of delirium. Collateral information from a reliable informant regarding the baseline cognitive functioning can help the differential. Delirium, unlike dementia, is often reversible, although in terminally ill patients, as noted previously, it may not be.

When Is Delirium Terminal in Nature?

At the last days or weeks of life, delirium may no longer be reversible due to the irreversible nature of the underlying medical etiologies. Delirium in terminally ill cancer patients is a relatively reliable predictor of approaching death in the coming days to weeks. In the palliative care setting, several studies support delirium reliably predicting impending death in patients with advanced cancer. Several prognostic tools for predicting survival in terminally ill cancer patients include delirium as a variable. Recognizing an episode of delirium, in the late phases of palliative care, is critically important in treatment planning and in advising family members about what to expect.

🔍 Key Point

When delirium corresponds with other forms of organ failure (e.g., liver, lung, or renal failure), a diagnosis of terminal delirium is most appropriate and informs the patient's prognosis and goals of care.

In terminally ill patients, the extent of diagnostic workup for and treatment of reversible causes of delirium is intrinsically linked to the goals of care. When assessing etiologies of delirium, an important challenge is the differentiation of delirium as either a reversible complication or an integral element of the dying process in terminally ill patients. When diagnostic information points to a likely etiology, specific therapy may be able to reverse delirium. However, the set of reversible etiologies of delirium may be limited by overall prognosis and goals of care. There is an ongoing debate as to the appropriate extent of diagnostic evaluation that should be pursued in a terminally ill patient with delirium. When confronted with delirium in terminally ill patients, the clinician must take an individualized and judicious approach, consistent with the goals of care. Care must be taken to select only diagnostic studies which do not incur excessive discomfort, and those for which the results may be actionable by employing treatments consistent with the goals of care. An etiology is discovered in about 40% of terminally ill patients with delirium, and about one-third to half of the patients with delirium improve with treatment of the specific etiologies. Reversibility of delirium is most associated with opioids, other psychoactive medications, and dehydration. Irreversibility of delirium is associated with hypoxic encephalopathy and metabolic factors related to major organ failure, including hepatic and renal insufficiency, and refractory hypercalcemia.

Clinical Management

The standard approach to managing delirium in palliative care settings, even in those with advanced disease, includes a search for underlying causes, correction of those factors, and management of the symptoms of delirium. Treatment of the symptoms of delirium should be initiated before, or concurrent with, a diagnostic assessment of the etiologies to minimize distress to patients, staff, and family members. The desired and often achievable outcome is a patient who is awake, alert, calm, comfortable, cognitively intact, and communicating coherently with family and staff.

Since publication of the American Psychiatric Association (APA) guidelines for treatment of delirium in 1999, a number of systematic reviews and guidelines have been released based on evidence-based management of delirium. In 2014, the American Geriatrics Society and the American College of Surgeons jointly released clinical practice guidelines for the prevention and treatment of postoperative delirium in older adults. The guidelines highlight the importance of multicomponent nonpharmacologic prevention strategies, education of healthcare professionals, medical evaluation of delirium etiology, optimizing pain management with nonopioids, and avoiding high-risk medications. The guidelines included avoidance of drug treatment for hypoactive delirium and avoidance of benzodiazepines for the treatment of delirium, except in cases of alcohol or benzodiazepine withdrawal.

In the terminally ill patient who develops delirium during the last days of life, the management of delirium is unique, presenting a number of dilemmas, and the desired clinical outcome may be significantly altered by the dying process. The goal of care in the terminally ill may shift to providing comfort through the judicious use of sedatives, even at the expense of alertness.

Pharmacological Treatments

Very often, nonpharmacologic interventions and supportive measures alone are often not effective in controlling the symptoms of delirium in palliative care settings. Symptomatic treatment with psychotropic medications is often essential to control the symptoms of delirium, although there are not any Food and Drug Administration (FDA) approved medications for this treatment of delirium.

APA provided guidance for the use of antipsychotics in the treatment of delirium in 1999. Antipsychotic use has since been studied in many settings and different patient populations in the last two decades (see Table 5.3).

Treatment with antipsychotic agents has been the norm in the everyday management of delirium across settings and different patient populations for more than two decades. Last decade has seen a surge in treatment trials in delirium.[11–15] Several recent studies did not show a clear benefit of antipsychotics in decreasing the duration or severity of delirium. Management of delirium in palliative care settings is nuanced and the goals of care must be central to pharmacological decision-making.

Short-term use of low-dose antipsychotics continues to be the mainstay of treatment for symptoms of delirium (e.g., severe agitation, delusions, and hallucinations interfering with care), with the understanding that antipsychotics are not expected to cure the underlying etiologies or to prolong survival, but to allow for patients to safely and successfully be managed and to ameliorate patient, staff, and caregiver distress, especially during the dying process. In the light of the recent research on use of antipsychotics, it is important

Table 5.3 Antipsychotic Medications in the Treatment of Delirium				
Medication	Initial Dose Range in the Terminally Ill	Routes of Administration	Side Effects	Comments
Typical antipsychotics				
Haloperidol	0.25–2 mg every 2–12 hr	PO, IV, IM, SC, syringe drivers*	Extrapyramidal adverse effects can occur at higher doses Monitor QTc interval on ECG depending on the goals of care	Remains the gold-standard therapy for delirium May add lorazepam (0.5–1 mg every 2–4 hr) for agitated patients
Chlorpromazine	12.5–50 mg every 4–6 hr	PO, IV, IM, SC, PR	More sedating and anticholinergic compared with haloperidol Monitor blood pressure for hypotension	May be preferred in agitated patients due to its sedative effect
Atypical antipsychotics				
Olanzapine	1.25–5 mg every 12–24 hr	PO,** IM	Sedation is the main dose-limiting adverse effect in short-term use	Older age, preexisting dementia, and hypoactive subtype of delirium have been associated with poor response
Risperidone	0.125–1 mg every 12–24 hr	PO**	Extrapyramidal adverse effects can occur with doses >2 mg/day Orthostatic hypotension	Clinical experience suggests better results in patients with hypoactive delirium
Quetiapine	12.5–50 mg every 12–24 hr	PO	Sedation, orthostatic hypotension	Sedating effects may be helpful in patients with sleep-wake cycle disturbance
Ziprasidone	10–20 mg every 12–24 hr	PO, IM	Monitor QT interval on ECG	Has not been found to be effective in controlling symptoms of delirium in ICU settings.
Aripiprazole	2–5 mg every 24 hr	PO,** IM	Monitor for akathisia	Evidence is limited to case reports, case series, and open label trials. Clinical experience suggests better results with hypoactive delirium.

*Syringe drivers are continuous subcutaneous infusions that can be used in the terminally ill patients in palliative care settings to allow for continuous symptom control and combination of multiple supportive medications.
**Risperidone, olanzapine, and aripiprazole are available in orally disintegrating tablets.
abbreviations: ECG, electrocardiogram; IM, intramuscular; IV, intravenous; PO, per oral; PR, per rectum; SC, subcutaneous.

to emphasize that in hypoactive delirium lacking symptoms interfering with management, or delirium of all subtypes that is mild to moderate severity, antipsychotics are best avoided or only used if the benefits of medications clearly outweigh the risks associated with their use.

Haloperidol (a "typical" antipsychotic) remains the gold-standard medication for treatment of symptoms of delirium among cancer patients, due to its efficacy in managing symptoms of delirium, and its safety. Haloperidol has few anticholinergic effects, lacks active metabolites, and is formulated for several routes of administration. In many parts of the world, haloperidol will be delivered continuously in subcutaneous low dosage via a syringe driver, often in combination with midazolam. Haloperidol, used at dosages lower than those commonly used in medically healthy adults (1–3 mg per day), is usually effective in targeting agitation and psychotic symptoms. In general medical and psychiatric settings, doses of haloperidol need not exceed 20 mg in a 24-hour period; however, some clinicians advocate higher doses in selected cases.

Lorazepam: In severe agitation related to delirium and in terminal delirium, clinicians may add lorazepam to haloperidol. This combination may be more effective in rapidly sedating patients and may help minimize any extrapyramidal adverse effects of haloperidol. There is evidence that benzodiazepines can worsen delirium; however, in palliative care settings, the combination of haloperidol with lorazepam/midazolam resulted in greater reduction in agitation compared to haloperidol alone. Where there is concern that lorazepam is worsening symptoms of delirium, switching to monotherapy with a more sedating antipsychotic, such as olanzapine or chlorpromazine, is an option.

The FDA has issued a warning about the risk of QTc prolongation and torsades de pointes with IV haloperidol. Thus, monitoring QTc intervals daily among medically ill patients receiving IV haloperidol has become the standard clinical practice.

Chlorpromazine: Oral or intravenous (IV) chlorpromazine is considered to be an effective alternative to haloperidol (with or without lorazepam) when increased sedation is required, especially in the ICU setting in the United States, where close blood pressure monitoring is feasible, and for severe agitation in terminally ill patients to decrease distress for the patient, family, and staff. It is important to monitor chlorpromazine's anticholinergic and hypotensive side effects, particularly in elderly patients. In many countries of the world, **levomepromazine** will be used as an alternative phenothiazine to chlorpromazine, especially in syringe drivers which are covered to avoid degradation by light.

"Atypical" antipsychotic agents (i.e., risperidone, olanzapine, quetiapine, ziprasidone, and aripiprazole) are increasingly used in the treatment of delirium due to decreased risk of extrapyramidal adverse symptoms (EPS).

Risperidone: this may be used in the treatment of delirium, starting at doses ranging from 0.125 to 1 mg and titrated up as necessary with particular attention to the risks of EPS, QTc prolongation, orthostatic hypotension, and sedation at higher doses.

Olanzapine: this can be started between 1.25 and 5 mg nightly (using buccal wafer, oral tablet or subcutaneous/intramuscular administration) and titrated up with sedation being the major limiting factor, although this may be favorable in the treatment of hyperactive delirium, where twice daily divided dosing may be used.

Quetiapine: start at a low dose of 12.5–50 mg and titrate up to 100–200 mg a day (usually at twice daily divided doses). Sedation and orthostatic hypotension are the main dose-limiting factors.

Aripiprazole: Limited evidence supports the use of the less sedating aripiprazole, especially in hypoactive delirium. Findings to-date and our clinical experience suggest a starting dose of 2 to 5 mg daily for aripiprazole, with a maximum dose of 15 mg daily.

Important considerations in starting treatment with any antipsychotic for delirium (see Figure 5.1) include EPS risk, sedation, anticholinergic side effects, cardiac arrhythmias, particularly prolonged QTc interval, and drug-drug interactions. Importantly, the FDA issued a "black box" warning of increased risk of death associated with the use of typical and atypical antipsychotics in elderly patients with dementia-related psychoses. Maintaining the QTc interval at <500 mms is desirable for safety.

Some clinicians have suggested that the hypoactive subtype of delirium may respond to psychostimulants such as methylphenidate and amphetamine, or to combinations of antipsychotics and psychostimulants, or

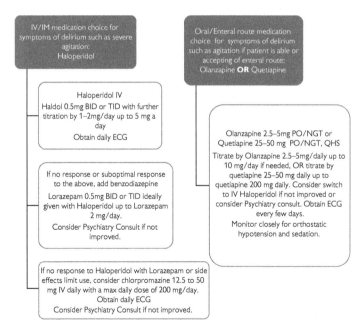

Figure 5.1 Decision tree for antipsychotic use in palliative care settings.

antipsychotics and wakefulness agents such as modafinil. However, studies with psychostimulants in treating delirium remain limited to case reports and open-label studies. The risks of precipitation or exacerbation of agitation or psychotic symptoms should be carefully evaluated when psychostimulants are considered in the treatment of delirium.

Dexmedetomidine: This alpha-2 agonist, mostly studied for use post-operatively and in critical care settings, has been compared to standard sedatives such as midazolam and propofol, to opioids, and to placebo, in randomized controlled trials. A systematic review and meta-analysis, with incidence and duration of delirium as the primary outcomes, showed that the administration of dexmedetomidine was associated with significantly lower overall incidence and duration of delirium when compared to placebo, propofol, midazolam, and opioids. The main side effects were increased risk of bradycardia and hypotension. It is important to emphasize that dexmedetomidine is used intravenously in postsurgical and critical care settings, and primarily for mechanically ventilated patients. Evidence for its use in palliative care settings remains limited; however, a 2021 open label trial supports further study of dexmedetomidine for hyperactive delirium in a palliative care setting by a continuous subcutaneous infusion route.

Social, Environmental, and Psychological Care

To date, most nonpharmacological delirium treatment research has occurred outside of a palliative care setting. The limited body of evidence does not support nonpharmacologic interventions for treatment of delirium in palliative care settings. Nevertheless, promising studies in other settings, a strong evidence base supporting a multicomponent nonpharmacological intervention to prevent delirium, and the low-risk nature of these interventions have led to the recommendation of their use for treatment as well as prevention of delirium. Box 5.3 includes a summary of commonly used nonpharmacological multicomponent delirium interventions.

Family Care

Both hypoactive and hyperactive subtypes of delirium have been shown to cause distress in family members, clinicians, and staff. Studies suggest the experience of caring for a delirious family member or a patient is perhaps even more of a distressing experience than the experience of the patient, may induce symptoms of anxiety and depression, and may persist for at least 12 months following the delirious episode. Clinicians may mitigate this distress by facilitating communication and by emphasizing aspects of the caregiver relationship that remain intact, in addition to managing symptoms of delirium. Family members should be encouraged to take breaks, possibly rotating the family member at the bedside to ensure respite and reduce caregiver distress. Family members may express concern when agitation or psychotic symptoms emerge in the context of delirium, e.g., "Did s/he lose her mind?" It is prudent for clinicians to explain the symptoms of delirium, its potential etiologies and commonality, as well as the management options. Most family members would view antipsychotic medications used to manage symptoms of delirium as "the treatment" of delirium. The clinicians should inform families that the

<header>CHAPTER 5 Delirium and Cognitive Impairment</header>

Box 5.3 Nonpharmacological Interventions for Delirium

✓ **Address cognitive impairment,** orient patient frequently, use a bulletin board with orienting information including the date, the room number, names of the medical team members.

✓ **Avoid dehydration and constipation** by ensuring adequate fluid intake

✓ **Assess for and manage hypoxia**

✓ **Look for and treat infection**, avoid unnecessary catheterization, and implement infection-control procedures.

✓ **Address immobility** or limited mobility

✓ **Assess for pain** via nonverbal signs, particularly in persons with communication difficulties, and initiate/review appropriate pain management.

✓ Carry out **a medication review** considering both the type and number of medications.

✓ **Address poor nutrition** and provide nutrition support. Ensure that dentures fit properly.

✓ **Address sensory impairment**. Resolve reversible cause of the impairment. Ensure hearing and visual aids are available to and used by persons who need them.

✓ **Promote good sleep** patterns and sleep hygiene. Avoid procedures during sleeping hours, schedule medication rounds to avoid disturbing sleep and reduce noise to a minimum.

✓ Adequate but not excessive **sensory stimulation**

✓ Low level **background light** at night

✓ Where possible **family presence**—comforting

✓ **Close observation** to ensure safety

---

antipsychotics control the symptoms of delirium, while treatment of the underlying etiologies would bring about the actual treatment of delirium. The short-term, low-dose use of antipsychotics should also be emphasized when providing education to caregivers, to not lead them into thinking these medications would be for long-term use.

Controversies in the Management of Terminal Delirium

The use of antipsychotics and other pharmacologic agents in the management of delirium in the dying patient remains controversial. Some researchers have argued that pharmacologic interventions are inappropriate in the dying patient. Delirium is viewed by some as a natural part of the dying process that should not be altered. Clearly, there are many patients who experience hallucinations and delusions during delirium that are pleasant and in fact comforting, and many clinicians may justifiably question the appropriateness of intervening pharmacologically in such instances. Another concern is that these patients are so close to death that aggressive treatment is unnecessary, and antipsychotics or sedatives may be inappropriately avoided because of exaggerated fears that they might hasten death through hypotension or respiratory depression.

Clinical experience in managing delirium in dying patients suggests that the use of antipsychotics in the management of agitation, paranoia, hallucinations, and altered sensorium is safe, effective, and often quite appropriate. Management of delirium on a case-by-case basis is most prudent. The agitated, delirious dying patient can be given antipsychotics to help restore calm. A "wait-and-see" approach may be appropriate with some patients who have a lethargic or somnolent presentation of delirium or who are having frankly pleasant or comforting hallucinations. Such a wait-and-see approach must, however, be tempered by the knowledge that a lethargic or hypoactive delirium may very quickly and unexpectedly become an agitated or hyperactive delirium that can threaten the serenity and safety of the patient, family, and staff. It is important to remember that, by their nature, the symptoms of delirium are unstable and fluctuate over time.

Perhaps the most challenging clinical problem is the management of the dying patient with a terminal delirium that is unresponsive to standard pharmacologic interventions. Approximately 30% of dying patients with delirium do not have their symptoms adequately controlled by antipsychotic medications. The addition of benzodiazepines to haloperidol appears to control agitation better in the setting of terminal delirium than haloperidol alone. Palliative sedation may be performed in terminally ill patients to manage one or more refractory symptoms. About a quarter to a third of all terminally ill patients undergo proportionate palliative sedation. The most frequent refractory adverse effects are delirium and dyspnea. The most widely used drugs for palliative sedation are midazolam and haloperidol for refractory delirium, but chlorpromazine/levomepromazine or other neuroleptics are also effective. When patients experience refractory symptoms during the last hours or days of life, palliative sedation using a syringe driver is a medical intervention aimed at managing the suffering.[16] Clinicians are sometimes concerned that the use of sedating medications may hasten death via respiratory depression, hypotension, or even starvation. However, studies have found that the use of opioids and psychotropic agents in hospice and palliative care settings is associated with longer rather than shorter survival. Palliative sedation in terminal cancer patients is feasible in both home and inpatient hospice settings.

The clinician must always keep in mind the goals of care and communicate these goals with staff, patients, and family members when treating delirium in the terminally ill. The clinician must weigh competing clinical imperatives when deciding how to best manage the dying patient with delirium in a manner that preserves and respects the dignity and values of the patient and family.

Prevention of Delirium

Most of the delirium prevention focus is on early detection, with risk models to predict those patients at risk for developing delirium, and pharmacological and nonpharmacological interventions being used to minimize risk of development of delirium symptoms.

Research into prevention of delirium in the ICU setting has identified sedative and analgesic use, age, educational attainment, hypertension history, alcohol use disorder history, prior history of delirium and elevation of Acute Physiology, Age, Chronic Health Evaluation II (APACHE-II) scores as risk factors for delirium. Use of physical restraints has also been identified as an independent risk factor for delirium persistence at the time of hospital discharge. Physical restraints should be avoided in all patients with delirium or at risk for delirium. To date, several risk models have been proposed for predicting those at risk for delirium in the ICU setting, however whether they have any value within a palliative care setting is not yet known.

Researchers have studied both pharmacologic and nonpharmacologic interventions in the prevention of delirium among older patient populations, particularly in surgical settings. The applicability of these interventions to the prevention of delirium in palliative care settings has not been widely studied. A 2016 Cochrane review examined prophylactic antipsychotics for preventing delirium in hospitalized non-ICU medical and surgical patients 16 years or older and found no clear evidence of an effect of antipsychotics on the incidence of delirium. The same review and meta-analysis found that there is no evidence to support the use of melatonin or ramelteon in reducing the incidence of delirium. On the other hand, it is common practice to use melatonin or melatonin agonists preferentially for insomnia in hospital settings to minimize the risk of delirium compared to the heightened risk of delirium associated with the use of other medications for sleep induction or maintenance (e.g., benzodiazepines, antihistamines).

Prevention of delirium with multicomponent nonpharmacologic approaches has been shown to be effective and has gained widespread acceptance as the most effective strategy for delirium.[17,18] Multicomponent nonpharmacological approaches studied include individualized care, use of checklists/protocols, education/training, reorientation, attention to sensory deprivation, nutrition/hydration, electrolytes, oxygenation, and identification of infection, mobilization, sleep hygiene, multidisciplinary team-based care, pain control, familiar objects, cognitive stimulation, medication review, mood assessment for anxiety/depression, bowel/bladder care, and management of postoperative complications. We advocate for a common-sense approach to implementing multicomponent nonpharmacological interventions in the setting of terminal illness, guided by the goals of care, and with recognition that many of these interventions are low risk and are likely to have benefits well beyond the endpoint of incidence of delirium, even in palliative care settings.

Case Study

Hadley is a 29-year-old woman with a left frontal IDH-wild type glioblastoma multiforme (GBM). Following surgical resection, Hadley was started on levetiracetam for seizure prophylaxis and on dexamethasone for cerebral edema at the postsurgical site. On postoperative day 2, psychiatry received an immediate consult request at 3:00 a.m. for Hadley trying to leave the hospital against medical advice. Security and nursing were by the elevators, trying to prevent the patient from leaving the hospital when the psychiatry fellow arrived. On assessment, Hadley presented with severe psychomotor agitation, pressured speech, disorientation, and poor recall of recent events. Haloperidol 1 mg intramuscularly was administered with good effect. Hadley walked back to her room with staff. She was reoriented to her room and the recent events. Her husband was notified, who stayed on the phone with her until his arrival at the hospital, reassuring her that she was safe in the hospital. On further assessment, Hadley was noted to be holding her head, and only when asked did she verbalize headache and pain at the surgical site. She was given analgesics. She was also started on quetiapine 25 mg nightly for insomnia, agitation, and paranoia. Dexamethasone taper was initiated. On postoperative day 7, Hadley was almost at her baseline with significant improvements in cognition, behavior, and sleep-wake cycle. Quetiapine was discontinued. Psychoeducation on delirium was provided to Hadley and her husband, who were highly distressed due to the delirium experience. An outpatient psychiatry follow-up appointment was scheduled to monitor cognition and help the patient cope with anxiety symptoms in the aftermath of her experience of delirium.

Professional Issues and Service Implementation

Recording and Communication Challenges

- Communication challenges are paramount in interacting with patients with delirium due to cognitive impairment and/or delusions that impair the ability to communicate effectively. Use of simple and short sentences, using verbal de-escalation techniques, and minimizing environmental stimuli may improve communication with the patients.
- Recording findings of delirium at the time of assessment is essential given the fluctuating nature of the syndrome. Patients with delirium are likely to present with different symptoms in the day and clear documentation of assessments at different time points would help any diagnostic clarification.
- Use of a delirium severity tool such as MDAS is encouraged to systematically record delirium severity longitudinally. This detailed recording would help with the judicious use of medications to treat symptoms of delirium. It would also unify all the teams involved in patient care with an objective measure in gauging improvements in delirium.
- An additional communication challenge for patients with delirium occurs when professional interpreters are needed. Phone interpreter services, most widely available in most hospital settings, fall short of providing benefit in facilitating communication in the setting of delirium. Most patients become increasingly confused, and even more paranoid with phone interpreter use. In-person professional interpreters are essential to most effectively communicate with these patients.

Legal Responsibilities

- Delirium and other cognitive syndromes may impact decision-making capacity in palliative care settings, where patients and families are likely to face important decisions regarding their care. Although advance care planning legislations may vary widely in different parts of the world, it is essential to identify surrogate decision makers early on. This would allow clinicians to turn to surrogates if the patient afflicted by cognitive impairment were not able to demonstrate capacity for decisions around delirium assessment and management, or more broadly goals of care discussions.

Common Ethical Dilemmas

- Delirium and other cognitive syndromes present a myriad of ethical dilemmas for clinicians, patients, and families involved. Patient autonomy may be at stake due to impaired decision-making capacity. Despite the cognitive changes, patients may retain some capacity for many decisions they face, hence the clinicians should assess and maintain patient involvement to the extent that is possible. When patients with severe delirium are unable to engage in decision-making, clinicians must turn to surrogate decision makers, ensuring patient autonomy is exercised through those who are well informed of the patient's values, goals, and wishes and act in his or her best interest.

- The principles of beneficence and nonmaleficence are constantly at play in palliative care settings. When facing decisions around the extent of diagnostic testing to discover etiologies of delirium, one must weigh risks versus benefits of the testing and how this may affect any suffering of the patient. Delirium in palliative care settings even in the last days to weeks of life may be due to reversible etiologies. An open discussion with the patient or the surrogates involved will help to determine how far to test and how much to treat, while always comforting.

- The principle of justice (e.g., access and equitable distribution of health resources) is the most debatable and variable ethical principle depending on what part of the world patients live. The availability of resources, size of the population, and the country's healthcare system all play a role in how this principle is taken into consideration.

Policies for Clinical Services

- Recognition of delirium remains a challenge in healthcare settings. Some hospitals have established policies around screening, assessment, and management of delirium that involve multiple disciplines, including but not limited to general medicine, geriatrics, nursing, and psychiatry. The buy-in from hospital administrators is essential for policies alike to be established. The growing literature on morbidity, hospital costs, and mortality associated with delirium and cognitive syndromes help advocate for the resources that are needed to develop such policies and programs.

Teams and Supervision Challenges

- An interdisciplinary approach is essential for the management of patients with delirium and other cognitive syndromes in palliative care settings. Nursing plays a pivotal role. Being at the bedside, observing the fluctuations in any symptoms of delirium, and closely interacting with families, nursing is in the best position to screen for delirium and to implement the nonpharmacological interventions for delirium prevention and treatment. Inpatient rounds should include interdisciplinary team members to allow for discussion of challenging cases, to educate staff on delirium, and to empower all with strategies to assess for and manage delirium.

- For psychiatrists and palliative care clinicians involved, the most important components of the liaison work are educating nursing and the medical teams about the nature of delirium, advocating for ongoing assessment of etiologies when indicated, or facilitating goals of care conversations when delirium points to worsening prognosis.

Physical therapists, occupational therapists, nursing, chaplains, clinical psychologists, and social workers can be a part of the delirium assessment and management team, especially in palliative care settings, where an interdisciplinary approach to care is of utmost importance to alleviate the suffering of patients and families.

References

1. Alici Y, Breitbart B. Delirium. In Breitbart W, et al., Editors. Psycho-Oncology. 4th ed. New York: Oxford University Press; 2021. Section VII, pages 345–354.

2. Inouye SK, Westendorp RGJ, Saczynski JS. Delirium in elderly people. Lancet. 2014;383(9920):911–922. https://doi.org/10.1016/S0140-6736(13)60688-1

3. Bush SH, Tierney S, Lawlor PG. Clinical assessment and management of delirium in the palliative care setting. Drugs. 2017;77(15):1623–1643. https://doi.org/10.1007/s40265-017-0804-3.

4. Hosie A, Davidson PM, Agar M, Sanderson CR, Phillips J. Delirium prevalence, incidence, and implications for screening in specialist palliative care inpatient settings: A systematic review. Palliat Med. 2012;27(6):486–498. doi:10.1177/0269216312457214.

5. Watt CL, Momoli F, Ansari MT, et al. The incidence and prevalence of delirium across palliative care settings: A systematic review. Palliat Med. 2019;33(8):865–877. https://doi.org/10.1177/0269216319854944.

6. Boettger S, Breitbart W. Delirium in supportive and palliative care. Palliat Support Care. 2021;19(3):267.

7. Edelstein A, Alici Y. Diagnosing and managing delirium in cancer patients. Oncology (Williston Park). 2017;31(9):686–III.

8. Maldonado JR. Delirium pathophysiology: An updated hypothesis of the etiology of acute brain failure. Int J Geriatric Psychiatry. 2017;33(11):1428–1457. doi:10.1002/gps.4823

9. Featherstone I, Hosie A, Siddiqi N, et al. The experience of delirium in palliative care settings for patients, family, clinicians and volunteers: A qualitative systematic review and thematic synthesis. Palliat Med. 2021;35(6):988–1004. Palliat Med. 10.1177/02692163211006313.

10. Finucane AM, Lugton J, Kennedy C, Spiller JA. The experiences of caregivers of patients with delirium, and their role in its management in palliative care settings: An integrative literature review. Psychooncology. 2017;26(3):291–300. Palliat Med. 10.1002/pon.4140.

11. Breitbart W, Alici Y. Evidence-based treatment of delirium in patients with cancer. J Clin Oncol. 2012;30(11):1206–1214. https://doi.org/10.1200/JCO.2011.39.8784.

12. Neufeld KJ, Yue J, Robinson TN, Inouye SK, Needham DM. Antipsychotic medication for prevention and treatment of delirium in hospitalized adults: A systematic review and meta-analysis. J Am Geriatr Soc. 2016;64(4):705–714. https://doi.org/10.1111/jgs.14076.

13. Finucane AM, Jones L, Leurent B, et al. Drug therapy for delirium in terminally ill adults. Cochrane Database of Systematic Reviews. 2020;(1). https://doi.org/10.1002/14651858.CD004770.pub3.

14. Nikooie R, Neufeld KJ, Oh ES, et al. Antipsychotics for treating delirium in hospitalized adults. Annals of Internal Medicine. 2019;171(7):485. https://doi.org/10.7326/m19-1860.

15. Burry L, Mehta S, Perreault MM, et al. Antipsychotics for treatment of delirium in hospitalised non-ICU patients. Cochrane Database of Systematic Reviews. 2018(6). doi:10.1002/14651858.CD005594.pub3.

16. Arantzamendi M, Belar A, Payne S, et al. Clinical aspects of palliative sedation in prospective studies. A systematic review. J Pain Symptom Manage. 2021;61(4):831–844.e10. https://doi.org/10.1016/j.jpainsymman.2020.09.022.

17. Martinez F, Tobar C, Hill N. Preventing delirium: Should non-pharmacological, multicomponent interventions be used? A systematic review and meta-analysis of the literature. Age and Ageing. 2014;44(2):196–204. https://doi.org/10.1093/ageing/afu173.

18. Siddiqi N, Harrison JK, Clegg A, et al. Interventions for preventing delirium in hospitalised non-ICU patients. Cochrane Database of Systematic Reviews. 2016. https://doi.org/10.1002/14651858.cd005563.pub3

Further Reading

Agar M, Bush SH. Delirium at the end of life. Med Clin North Am. 2020;104(3):491–501. https://doi.org/10.1016/j.mcna.2020.01.006. An excellent review on delirium at the end of life.

American Geriatrics Society Expert Panel on Postoperative Delirium in Older Adults. American Geriatrics Society, abstracted clinical practice guideline for postoperative delirium in older adults. J Am Geriatr Soc. 2015;63(1):142–150. https://doi.org/10.1111/jgs.13281. Guidelines with focus on older adults with postoperative delirium

Bush SH, Lawlor PG, Ryan K, et al. Delirium in adult cancer patients: ESMO Clinical Practice Guidelines. Ann Oncol. 2018;29 Suppl 4:iv143–iv165. https://doi.org/10.1093/annonc/mdy147. A thorough review of delirium in cancer patients.

Lawlor PG, Rutkowski NA, MacDonald AR, et al. A scoping review to map empirical evidence regarding key domains and questions in the clinical pathway of delirium in palliative care. J Pain Symptom Manage. 2019;57(3):661–681.e12. doi:10.1016/j.jpainsymman.2018.12.002. A comprehensive review of the existing literature on delirium in palliative care settings.

Meagher D, Agar MR, Teodorczuk A. Debate article: Antipsychotic medications are clinically useful for the treatment of delirium. Internat J Geriat Psychiat. 2017;33(11):1420–1427. https://doi.org/10.1002/gps.4759. Excellent article reviewing pros and cons of antipsychotic medications in the treatment of delirium from two different perspectives.

Chapter 6

Diagnosing Dying and Assessing Death Wishes

Cristina Monforte-Royo, Josep Porta-Sales, and Albert Balaguer

Learning Objectives

After reading this chapter, the clinician will be able to:

1. Recognize the signs of imminent death as the disease progresses and frailty develops.
2. Become skilled in psychological and pharmacological support for a dying patient.
3. Have an understanding of issues in communicating about imminent death to the patient and broader family.
4. Be able to assess, manage, and reassure patients regarding symptom control including support of fear of death and any other anxieties.
5. Understand the phenomenon of, and factors associated with, the wish to hasten death (WTHD) in the context of patients with advanced illness.
6. Be skilled in the clinical assessment and use of different instruments for assessing the WTHD.
7. Be aware of key issues in caring for the dying, including ethical, legal, training, and service development needs.

Background Evidence

Diagnosing Dying in Patients with Advanced Illness

How can clinicians predict and communicate that the patient has entered the dying phase of illness? Although the timing of death is difficult to predict, the majority of deaths associated with chronic and/or progressive illnesses like cancer are usually preceded by a period of clinical and functional deterioration. This provides time to prepare for death at all levels—biophysiologically, psychologically, socially, spiritually, and existentially.

The need to predict an imminent death is vital. Patients and families usually ask for the prognosis and/or an estimation of when death will occur.[1] This information is key to much planning about care provision. However, to predict if a patient is actively dying is not an easy task.[2] Recent studies show that clinical teams do not recognize the dying phase well, with a range of precision of survival estimates between 23% and 78%.[3] Numerous studies support the concern of clinicians and researchers who seek a "good death" or "good dying process."[4,5] However, this is greatly aided by accurate prognostication.

Even though there are diverse prognostic tools used in palliative care,[6] no studies exist that implement these tools in a systematic way, and the most used method is an actual clinical evaluation of the patient. The European Association for Palliative Care (EAPC) maintains that this clinical prediction is a valid method to obtain a general idea of prognosis, despite the limitations of interobserver variability. For that reason, use of prognostic tools that include the evaluation of clinical signs such as functional status, anorexia-cachexia, dyspnea, cognitive decline, or delirium is recommended. Information can be complemented by lab analyses (leukocytosis, lymphocytopenia, elevated C-reactive protein) to prognosticate the end of life.

Clinicians tend to overestimate or underestimate survival.[3] However, greater precision exists toward the last two weeks of life or near death, because clinicians in palliative care assess and reassess signs of imminent death with higher frequency.

The *Oxford Textbook of Palliative Medicine*[7] defines the terminal phase as "the period of inexorable and irreversible decline in functional status before death." The terminal phase or the phase of imminent death lasts from 24 hours to ≈14 days. This terminal phase has three stages, which can be seen in Box 6.1, which includes the most frequent signs and symptoms.

As well as the difficulty diagnosing imminent death effectively,[3] clinicians may also avoid talking about death and dying with patients and families. Communication within the team helps in planning and communication with the patient and family and is key to implementing optimal care to achieve a "good death."

Acceptance of Dying as a Normal Psychological Process

Acceptance of dying is an active process wherein the patient becomes open to and acknowledges his or her situation, whether physically or emotionally, to make the most of the time he or she has left. To accept that you are dying is not easy. Not all patients want to know they are near death; although recent studies show that the majority would like to have an opportunity to talk about the end of life, and they appreciate the benefits of doing so.[5] One systematic review showed that patients wish to know their prognosis when they are in the initial phases of cancer; however, evidence from patients with advanced illness or at end of life is scarce.

Terminally ill patients do not always accept the closeness of death, and many require mental healthcare to manage the negative emotions generated by the awareness of their mortality. Acceptance of dying is more commonly found in those that feel they have fulfilled their social roles and lived a life full of meaning; others may use a modest level of denial to cope. Recognition and acceptance of a life lived as well as possible becomes a worthy goal for many. Nevertheless, the experience of dying differs for each person. Recognition of

---

Box 6.1 Signs of Imminent Death

Syndrome of Imminent Death
Practically all patients at the end of life go through a pattern of signs and symptoms in the days before death. This trajectory often is called "active dying" or "imminent death."

Stages
- Early
  - Bed bound
  - Loss of interest and/or loss of ability to drink/eat
  - Cognitive changes: increasing time spent sleeping and/or delirium
- Middle
  - Further decline in mental status to obtundation (slow to arouse with stimulation; only brief periods of wakefulness)
- Late
  - Death rattle—pooled oral secretions that are not cleared due to loss of swallowing reflex
  - Coma
  - Fever—usually from aspiration pneumonia
  - Altered respiratory pattern—periods of apnea, hyperpnea, or irregular breathing
  - Mottled extremities

---

the dying trajectory empowers the best possible care for the patient and an opportunity to prepare family and significant others.

In Box 6.2, the guidelines of the National Consensus Project for Quality Palliative Care in the United States[8] suggests the following key elements of the quality of life of patients facing their death:

Box 6.2 Guidelines for Quality Care of the Dying and Their Families

- Signs and symptoms of impending death are recognized and communicated, and care appropriate for this phase of illness is provided to patient and family.
- Transition to the actively dying phase is recognized, when possible, and is documented and communicated appropriately to patient, family, and staff.
- End of life concerns, hopes, fears, and expectations are discussed openly and honestly in the context of social and cultural customs in a developmentally appropriate manner.
- Symptoms at the end of life are assessed and documented with appropriate frequency and are treated, based on patient/family preferences.

The Concept of the Desire for Hastened Death or Wish to Hasten Death

It is not uncommon for patients with advanced illness to experience a wish to hasten death (WTHD),* and this remains a source of concern for health professionals. To better understand this phenomenon, it is first necessary to clarify the concept. One of the first systematic reviews of the WTHD highlighted the lack of terminological precision in the literature,[9] leading the authors to propose a conceptual framework that sought to distinguish between generic thoughts about dying, the wish to die, and the intention to act on that wish. They went on to conduct a consensus study and proposed an international consensus statement (see Box 6.3) regarding the WTHD in the context of advanced illness.

A systematic review[11] of primary qualitative studies conducted in the United States, Canada, Australia, and China concluded that the WTHD is not only a reaction to suffering of multiple origins but also can mean different things to different patients, for whom it does not necessarily imply a genuine wish to bring an end to life.

We proposed an explanatory model of the WTHD among patients with advanced illness, comprising the following themes:

- the WTHD emerges in the context of physical, psychological, spiritual, and existential suffering;
- the loss of self, in the sense of a loss of function, of control, of meaning in life, or of perceived dignity; and
- fear, both of death itself and of the process of dying. In this situation, the patient can experience hopelessness and intense emotional distress.

Thus, the WTHD emerges as:

- The desire to live but not in this way,
- A way of ending suffering, and
- A kind of control, like having "an ace up one's sleeve just in case."

This model was updated later,[12] and five themes were identified:

1. Suffering as an experience common to all patients,
2. Reasons for the WTHD,
3. Meaning of the WTHD,

Box 6.3 Concept of Wish to Hasten Death*

The WTHD is a reaction to suffering, in the context of a life-threatening condition, from which the patient can see no way out other than to accelerate his or her death. This wish may be expressed spontaneously or after being asked about it, but it must be distinguished from the acceptance of impending death or from a wish to die naturally, although preferably soon. The WTHD may arise in response to one or more factors, including physical symptoms (either present or foreseen), psychological distress (e.g., depression, hopelessness, fears), existential suffering (e.g., loss of meaning in life), or social aspects (e.g., feeling that one is a burden).

*Adapted with permission from Balaguer et al.10

4. Functions of the WTHD, and
5. Lived experience of a timeline toward death and dying.

Overall, this new synthesis corroborated the aforementioned consensus statement on the WTHD, highlighting that it is a reaction to suffering that does not necessarily imply a genuine wish to die, but rather a wish to bring an end to suffering.

Mention should also be made of studies examining the WTHD from a quantitative perspective. One of the first, by Chochinov et al.,[13] found that the 8.5% of patients who expressed a WTHD were more likely to have symptoms of depression and low family support. Rosenfeld et al.[14] studied terminally ill cancer patients in the United States and found that 16.3% reported a strong wish to die. The WTHD was positively and significantly associated with depressive symptoms, hopelessness, poorer perceived quality of life, functional impairment, and physical symptoms. Further evidence from a study in Australia found that 14% of patients reported a high WTHD,[15] and that this was positively and significantly associated with a higher level of depressive symptoms, a greater perception of being a burden to others, and lower levels of social support. Finally, a study conducted in Spain found that 16.8% reported a high WTHD[16] and that this was positively and significantly associated with depressive symptoms, functional impairment, and dependency in relation to activities of daily living. Taken together, these four studies[13–16] suggest an overall prevalence of the WTHD between 8.5% and 16.8% among the 648 palliative care patients.

🔑 Key Points

Several studies that examined mediators and moderators of WTHD reported the following:

- Depression and hopelessness were independent predictors of the WTHD.[13,17]
- Depression and meaning in life were significant mediators of the relationship between functional impairment and the WTHD.[18]
- Depression and perceived loss of dignity have a direct effect while loss of control and functional impairment were antecedents and indirect precursors of the WTHD.[19]
- Loss of meaning and hopelessness were significant independent and synergistic factors in predicting high levels of WTHD. Breitbart and colleagues have studied how treating depression can eliminate the WTHD.[20]

The results of all these studies illustrate how the WTHD in patients with advanced illness is a complex phenomenon of multifactor origins that is best understood as a reaction to suffering, as proposed in the aforementioned consensus statement.

Presenting Problems

Symptoms and Signs Associated with Recognition of Dying or Imminent Death

The physiologic changes shown in Table 6.1 can help you to recognize when someone is entering the terminal phase or when someone is dying.

Table 6.1 Symptoms and Signs to Diagnose Dying

Physiologic Changes	Signs/Symptoms
General Changes	
Profound or extreme weakness, fatigue	Drowsy for extended periods
	Sleeping more
	Being less responsive and less able to communicate
	Getting worse day by day or hour by hour Becoming bed-bound for most of the day
	Needing help with all personal care
Disoriented with respect to time and a severely limited attention span.	More withdrawn and detached from surroundings May appear to be in a comatose-like state
Patient may speak to persons who have already died or see places others cannot see	Family may think these are hallucinations or a drug reaction
Delirium	Increased restlessness, confusion, and agitation
The person telling you they feel like they are dying	
Respiratory	
Retention of secretions in the pharynx and the upper respiratory tract.	Noisy respirations—usually no cough or weak cough
	Noisy chest secretions
Changes in their normal breathing pattern	
Dyspnea	Shortness of breath
Cheyne-Stokes respirations	Notable changes in breathing
Cardiac and Circulation Changes	
Decreased blood perfusion	Skin may become mottled and discolored Mottling and cyanosis of the upper extremities appear to indicate impending death versus such changes in the lower extremities
Decreased cerebral perfusion	Decreased level of consciousness or terminal delirium
	Drowsiness/disorientation
Decrease in cardiac output and intravascular volume	Tachycardia
	Hypotension
	Central and peripheral cyanosis and peripheral cooling.
Urinary and fecal function	
Decreased urinary output	Possible urinary incontinence Concentrated urine
	New urinary or fecal incontinence
Food and Fluids	
Decreased interest in food and fluid	Weight loss
	Dehydration

(continued)

Table 6.1 Continued

Physiologic Changes	Signs/Symptoms
Swallowing difficulties	Food pocketed in cheeks or mouth/choking with eating/coughing after eating
	Difficulty swallowing oral medication
Skin	
Skin may become mottled or discolored	Patches of purplish or dark pinkish color can be noted on back and posterior arms/legs
	Feeling cold to the touch
Decubitus ulcers may develop from pressure of being bedbound, decreased nutritional status	Red spots to bony prominences are first signs of Stage I decubiti, and open sores may develop

Key Challenges in Identifying Imminent Death

• To accurately identify the signs and symptoms of imminent death.
• To be trained in the use of prognostic tools.
• Training and expertise regarding care of patients nearing the end of life.
• Interdisciplinary teamwork that guarantees holistic care for the patient and family in the days before death.
• Communication between team members.
• Communication from the professionals with the patient and family about imminent death.

Symptoms and Signs Associated with the Wish to Hasten Death

• Functional impairment
• Loss of autonomy
• Physical symptoms: pain, nausea, general discomfort, weakness, fatigue, frailty
• Dependency
• Psychological symptoms: depression, hopelessness, anxiety, anhedonia, fear, perceived loss of dignity, fear of suffering, emotional distress
• Spiritual/existential issues: loss of meaning in life, dissatisfaction with or lack of purpose in life, not being at peace
• Social aspects: perception of being a burden to others, change in role (social, family, professional), loneliness, lack of social support, perception of being a financial burden
• The WTHD may emerge in response to one or more of these factors, which may be either already present or foreseen.

Key Challenges in Identifying a WTHD

• Availability of a suitable instrument (guide or tool) for exploring a possible WTHD, one that is able to distinguish the phenomenon and is useful and practical in the clinical context.
• Perception among clinicians that exploring the WTHD may be upsetting for, or harmful to, the patient.

- Clinicians may avoid exploring the WTHD for fear of not knowing how to respond to and manage it adequately.
- Need for clinical training to underpin the development of individualized and appropriate care plans for patients.
- Knowing when it is the best moment to proactively and routinely explore a possible WTHD among patients with advanced illness.

Key Differential Diagnoses

Key Differentials in the Imminent Death
- Inaccurate prognostication
- Indolent versus aggressive cancers
- Unpredictability of infection or acute events like stroke or cardiac events

Key Differentials in the Wish to Hasten death
- Depression: this should always be ruled out when a patient with advanced illness expresses a WTHD.
- Demoralization syndrome: existential distress in patients at the end of life, which includes symptoms of hopelessness and helplessness caused by a loss of purpose and meaning in life.
- Lack of social support.
- Poorly treated pain or other physical symptoms causing debility.

Assessment and Investigations

Predicting Imminent Death
As the EAPC suggests, the use of valid and reliable instruments helps to refine the diagnosis of imminent death.

According to the systematic review by Lau,[1] there are four non-disease-specific prognostic tools and four disease-specific prognostic tools in cancer used in palliative care (shown in Box 6.4).

Exploring the Wish to Hasten Death

The nature of the WTHD and the vulnerability of the population who experience it make studying the epidemiology of the phenomenon a challenge, one that is made even more difficult by the use of different instruments to assess this wish. With the aim of characterizing these instruments, our group conducted a systematic review of 50 studies that have sought to assess the WTHD using a measurement instrument or semistructured interview.[21] The review, whose goal was to identify these instruments and to rate their reported psychometric properties, found that five of the seven instruments identified had been designed for a specific study and had not, to date, been applied elsewhere. By contrast, the other two instruments have been widely

Box 6.4 Prognostic Tools Used in Palliative Care

Non-Disease-Specific Prognostic Tools

- Palliative Performance Scale (PPS): is a simple assessment tool for functional status that has been used to predict the range of survival from <1 week to 6 months. Lower PPS levels are associated with lower survival probability and shorter duration.

- Palliative prognostic score (PaP): it can be used to predict 30-day survival probability. It has been used in different settings. It requires the inclusion of symptoms and blood tests.

- Prognostic index for one-year mortality in older adults (PIMOA): it is appropriate for adults 70 years of age or older discharged from hospital following an acute medical illness. It is based on Activity of Daily Living (ADL) scores, comorbid conditions, and lab tests. It could be used to predict one-year mortality rates.

- Mortality risk index (MRIS): It is used for newly admitted nursing home residents. It is based on a subset of the minimum data set variables, and it can be used to predict one-year mortality rates.

Disease-Specific Prognostic Tools in Cancer

- Intrahospital cancer mortality risk model (ICMRM): estimates the probability of surviving a short-term hospital stay (median: 8 days) based on Eastern Cooperative Oncology Group (ECOG) score, emergency admission, and lab tests.

- Cancer prognostic scale (CPS): It is based on tumor sites, functions and symptoms. It can estimate short-term survival of up to two weeks for cancer patients staying in an inpatient palliative care service.

- Palliative Prognostic Index (PPI): It estimates survival of up to six weeks in different palliative care settings and is based on PPS and four symptoms.

- Lung cancer prognostic model (LCPM): It is used for community-based home hospice patients with end-stage lung cancer. It estimates survival times ranging from <3 days to >1 year based on the number of ADL factors, tumor sites, and symptoms.

used (in 45 of the 50 studies) internationally. These two instruments, shown in Box 6.5, are:

- Desire for Death Rating Scale (DDRS)
- Schedule of Attitudes toward Hastened Death (SAHD).

Given the considerable variability in the reported prevalence of the WTHD (3.3%–20% using the DDRS and 3.9%–28% with the SAHD), the authors of the aforementioned systematic review[21] point out that these figures should be interpreted with caution due to methodological differences between studies with regard to sample characteristics, the percentage of eligible patients who actually participated, or the study design itself. They also note that the DDRS is more geared toward the assessment of patients in

---

Box 6.5 Key Instruments to Assess a Wish to Hasten Death

Desire for Death Rating Scale

- A face valid semistructured interview
- It begins with a screening question, which, if endorsed, is followed by a further three questions
- The clinician rates the patient's responses on a scale of 0 to 6, and a score of 3 or higher is generally considered indicative of a strong wish to die
- Prevalence of WTHD in studies using the DDRS in palliative care patients with advanced disease ranges from 3.3% to 20%; specifically, prevalence ranges from 6.5% to 15% in studies that used a cut-off score of ≥3, and from 3.3% to 20% in those that used a cut-off ≥4.
- It has been used in patients with cancer
- Given its nature (face-to-face interview), it has not been empirically validated

Schedule of Attitudes toward Hastened Death

- Validated instrument, whose psychometric properties have been most often analyzed
- Original instrument in English
- Adapted for use in several languages (German, Greek, Korean, and Spanish)
- 20 true/false items
- It may be used as a self-report or clinician-administered tool
- The total score ranges from 0 to 20, and a score of 10 or higher has generally been considered to indicate a strong desire for hastened death.
- Prevalence of the hastened death in studies that have used the SAHD in palliative care patients with advanced disease ranges from 3.9% to 28% in studies that used a cut-off score of ≥7, from 4.6% to 17% in those that used a cut-off ≥10 and from 5% to 8.8% in those that employed a cut-off ≥11.

---

clinical practice, whereas the SAHD is best suited to research, given its length (20 items) and the fact that the direct wording of its items may make it less suitable for patients who are physically and/or emotionally fragile.

A further issue to consider, and one that is acknowledged by the authors of the SAHD, is the difficulty of discriminating between a genuine wish to die and simply the acceptance of death by patients at the end of life; it is because of this that they propose using a cut-off of ≥10 on the SAHD. These limitations notwithstanding, both the SAHD and the DDRS have become the most widely used instruments in the field.

A final point of note is that two short forms of the SAHD are now available: a 6-item version of the original scale in English and a 5-item Spanish version. In both cases, the short form yielded validity indices comparable to those of the original version.

A New Instrument for Assessing the Wish to Hasten Death in Clinical Practice

More recently, our group has proposed the AFEDD (Assessment of the Frequency and Extent of the Desire to Die),[22] a short semistructured interview for detecting and assessing the WTHD in clinical practice, as shown in Box 6.6.

To explore whether using the AFEDD to proactively assess the WTHD was acceptable to patients with advanced illness, we administered the AFEDD and also asked patients two questions:

• whether they found talking about a possible WTHD upsetting; and
• whether they considered it important to talk about it.

Among patients who did not report a WTHD ($n = 147$), 95.9% said they were not at all upset by being asked, 3.4% were somewhat upset, and only 1 patient found it quite upsetting. For patients who did report a WTHD, 89.1% said they were not at all upset by being asked, while the remaining 10.9% found it somewhat upsetting. When asked about the importance of talking or being asked about the WTHD, 79.6% of patients who did not report such a wish said that it was very or fairly important to do so. Among those who did report a WTHD, 80.4% felt that it was a very or fairly important issue to discuss. Notably, only one patient (who did not report a WTHD) considered that being asked about it was not important.

Clinical Management

Managing Dying

According to the *Clinical Practice Guidelines for Quality of Palliative Care*, as the patient approaches death, the comprehensive assessment and management of pain and physical symptoms, as well as attention to social, spiritual, psychological, and cultural aspects are of vital importance. This guideline, as well

---

Box 6.6 Interview to Assess the Wish to Hasten Death

Assessment of the Frequency and Extent of the Desire to Die

• Semistructured interview
• It begins with a screening question: "Some people in your situation may involuntarily start to think that living like this is not worth it anymore. Lately (in the last week or two), have you thought that living like this is not worth it?"
• If endorsed, the clinician follows up with two questions regarding the frequency and extent of the WTHD, which are rated on a scale from 1 to 4
• AFEDD total score ranges from 0 (if the screening question is not endorsed) to 8, with higher scores indicating a stronger WTHD.

as the *Oxford Textbook of Palliative Medicine*,[7] propose the need for care of the patient near imminent death with an interdisciplinary team to guarantee proper care. The team should include professionals with training in end of life care, in assessment and symptom management, and with appropriate skills to communicate with patients and families regarding the signs and symptoms of an imminent death.

Essentials of Care of the Patient in a Situation of Imminent Death

• To assess and control the most common physical symptoms in patients nearing their end, such as pain, dyspnea, nausea, agitation, delirium, and respiratory secretions.
• To ensure adequate contact with the patient and the family in the days prior to imminent death.
• To identify the signs and symptoms of impending death.
• To explore with the patient and family how they wish to approach the end of life.
• To identify spiritual concerns related to the process of dying and death.
• To facilitate, attend to, and adapt care to the cultural aspects and needs of the patient and family.
• To facilitate and propose legacy building, such as with life review, letters to friends and family, and even making a diary in video format.
• To facilitate resolution of any legal concerns.
• To coordinate care for patients and the importance of a transfer to the appropriate service for better care.
• To plan care both at the time of death and even after death.
• To prepare the family to know how to recognize the signs and symptoms of imminent death, as well as how to manage the symptoms.

Table 6.2 presents suggested activities for care focused on ensuring the comfort of the patient close to death, both pharmacological and nonpharmacological: Additionally, a multidisciplinary team should help to manage uncertainty and support the family with all their needs.

These activities in the care of the person close to death can be accompanied by complementary therapies.[23] There have been applications of music therapy, massage therapy,[24] mindfulness, and aromatherapy that are shown to have positive effects in the control of anxiety and distress. For spiritual care, some centers rely on chaplaincy services or pastoral care workers.

Managing the Wish to Hasten Death

A team of researchers and palliative care clinicians have developed a training course aimed at improving health professionals' self-confidence in responding to the patient's expression of a WTHD.[25] There was considerable consensus over the importance of proactively addressing the wish to die. Almost all of the patients who were interviewed saw the potential value, from an emotional perspective, in having such a conversation with a professional, even if they (the patient) did not currently experience a WTHD.

Table 6.2 Care Principles Close to Death

Physiologic Changes	Activities
Profound or extreme weakness, fatigue and weakness	This is normal. Educate family.
Disoriented with respect to time and a severely limited attention span.	This is normal. Educate family.
Patient may speak to persons who have already died or see places others cannot see.	If patient appears frightened, treat with medication. Otherwise, educate family that this is normal and common.
Delirium	Treat agitation with medication, mainly neuroleptics such as Haloperidol, but in some circumstances palliative sedation will be indicated.
The person telling you they feel like they are dying	It may be a good moment to talk about preferences of the place of dying. Facilitating saying goodbye to family and friends. Exploring and treating spiritual needs: chaplaincy, pastoral support, volunteers, etc.
Retention of secretions in the pharynx and the upper respiratory tract.	Adjust head of bed up to 45 degrees. Can fold small soft pillow or towel behind neck for extra support. Frequently, anticholinergic drugs are needed.
Changes in their normal breathing pattern	Educate family.
Dyspnea	Oxygen at 2–3 liters may help for some patients and often helps families to feel better. Increase in dose of opioids or benzodiazepines should also be considered.
Cheyne-Stokes respirations	A gentle fan blowing toward the patient may provide relief. Educate families that this is normal as the patient is dying.
Decreased blood perfusion	Provide good skin care. Turn patient every 2–3 hours if this does not cause discomfort. Lotion to back and extremities. Support extremities with soft pillows.
Decreased cerebral perfusion	Orient patient gently if tolerated and this is not upsetting. Allow patient to rest.
Decrease in cardiac output and intravascular volume	Comfort measures. Space out activities.
Decreased urinary output	Keep patient clean and dry. Place a Foley catheter if skin starts to break down or if patient is large and difficult to change diapers or if caregiver unable to provide diaper and linen changes.
Decreased interest in food and fluid.	Do not force fluid or foods. Provide excellent mouth care.

Table 6.2 Continued	
Physiologic Changes	**Activities**
Swallowing difficulties	Soft foods and thickened fluids as tolerated. Stop feeding patient if choking or pocketing food.
Skin may become mottled or discolored.	Keep sheets clean and dry. Avoid paper underpass directly against skin. Apply lotion as tolerated.
Decubitus ulcers may develop from pressure of being bedbound, decreased nutritional status.	Relieve pressure to bony prominences or other areas of breakdown with turning and positioning every 2 hr if tolerated. If patient has increased pain or discomfort with position changes, decrease the frequency. Special mattress as needed. Specialized skin patch to Stage I–II ulcers. Change each 5–7 days or as needed. Goals of wound care for Stage III and IV decubiti should be to promote comfort and prevent worsening rather than healing since healing most likely will not occur. Consider application of specialized products if smells are present.

With the aim of exploring how best to respond to a WTHD in clinical practice, we have synthesized guidelines and protocols into the following categories: the legal context, communication with the patient, aspects that the professional needs to be aware of, aspects to explore, the professional's communication skills and the professional's responsibilities. In Box 6.7, we summarize this approach for clinicians.

In terms of nonpharmacologic approaches, several psychotherapeutic approaches have been shown to decrease desire for hastened death—specifically, Meaning-Centered Psychotherapy by Breitbart et al.[26] Also, Chochinov et al.[27] developed dignity therapy or dignity-conserving end of life care, which has promoted a heightened sense of dignity, an increased sense of purpose, and the will to live.

In terms of pharmacologic approaches, the treatment of comorbidities such as depression, pain, breathlessness, nausea, and insomnia that can contribute to a WTHD have revealed interesting results. Breitbart et al.[20] demonstrated that pharmacologic treatment of comorbid depression in patients with AIDS and with cancer diminished the desire for hastened death. A recent study by Griffiths et al.[28] suggest that psilocybin-assisted psychotherapy may decrease symptoms of depression and anxiety for at least 6 months. Ross et al.[29] showed that psilocybin-assisted psychotherapy produced quick, substantial, and sustained improvements in anxiety and depression and led to decreases in cancer-related demoralization and hopelessness, improved spiritual well-being, and increased quality of life. In addition, various studies using ketamine in patients with advanced cancer have been shown to rapidly reduce suicidal ideation.[30]

Box 6.7 Management Principles in Caring for the Dying

- As the patient approaches death, the comprehensive assessment and management of pain and physical symptoms, social, spiritual, psychological, and cultural concerns, are of vital importance.
- Working in a multidisciplinary team helps greatly to care for the patient approaching death, including managing uncertainty and assisting family members.
- There exist various treatments, both pharmacological and nonpharmacological, to manage comorbidities related to approaching death and the WTHD.
- Complementary therapies can show benefits for psychospiritual care of the patient and the family.
- The WTHD among patients with advanced illness is complex, yet can be assessed and quantified.
- Physical, emotional, spiritual, existential and social factors, both present and foreseen, may all contribute to a WTHD.
- Use of assessment instruments of the WTHD can be easily incorporated into clinical practice, is beneficial, and doesn't upset patients.
- Patients consider it important to talk about a possible WTHD.
- Exploring the WTHD is an opportunity to understand it, to detect possibly hidden sources of suffering, and to seek to alleviate this suffering.

Professional Issues and Service Implementation

Ethical

Imminent Death

There is an ethical and professional commitment to care for the patient and their family throughout any anguish, striving for a peaceful death. The dying process impacts emotionally on the family and the care team, which can cause emotional exhaustion or burnout. The clinical team strives to prevent this and support the family. In any case, the team will be committed to ensuring that the family has adequate resources to cope with the distress of the events leading to and after death and to never give up.

Alternatively, there are countries where it is possible to establish advance directives (see Chapter 1), where the patient and family will talk about their preferences for treatment and place of death, medical power of attorney, and how they hope it will be a "good death."

The Wish to Hasten Death

Faced with a patient who expresses a WTHD, the primary ethical duty of health professionals is to listen to and accompany that person, and to do what they can to relieve his or her suffering. One of the first steps should be to rule out demoralization (see Chapter 3) and depression (see Chapter 4), with treatment being offered if necessary. However, it is also important to understand the meaning of the WTHD for individual patients, and to identify where the roots of their suffering lie. Thus, before interpreting the WTHD as a deliberate expression of personal autonomy, it is essential to explore all the possible factors—physical, psychological, and social, both present and foreseen—that may be contributing to the person's suffering, and hence to their wish to die. Many of these factors are likely to be amenable to intervention by the palliative care team, with additional input, as necessary, from other specialists. The patient's family can also play a key role in offering support, and it may occasionally be helpful to call on adequately trained volunteers to help the lonely and isolated.

Interventions and support systems of this kind should form the cornerstone of our response to patients with advanced illness who express a WTHD. If, as health professionals, we simply accept such a wish at face value, rather than exploring what lies behind it, we risk abandoning patients to their suffering, and hence we fail in our ethical duty to provide them with adequate care.

Cultural

Another aspect that is part of a quality dying process is the adaptation to culture and traditions of each person and family. Assessing and respecting values, beliefs, and traditions related to illness, death, family caregiver roles, and decision-making are the first steps in providing culturally sensitive palliative care. Different cultures have different traditions related to death and, when caring for patients belonging to a particular faith or culture (see Chapter 9), professionals should become familiar with the traditions that the patient and family would like to observe.

Legal

In some countries such as Netherlands, Belgium, Luxemburg, Colombia, Canada, and very recently Spain and New Zealand (by order of decriminalization), the practice of euthanasia is an option. There is also assisted suicide in these same countries (except Colombia), as well as in Switzerland, Australia, some states in the United States (California, Colorado, Hawaii, Maine, Montana, New Jersey, New Mexico, Oregon, Vermont, and Washington, and also Washington, DC). The Constitutional Courts of Germany, Austria, Colombia, and Italy have legalized assisted suicide, but their governments have not yet legislated or regulated this practice.

Box 6.8 shows the typical requirements to ensure the law is correctly applied, as legislated in most countries. Here we summarize the broad principles as details vary across jurisdictions. Generally, palliative care services offer their clinical care without getting involved in the provision of euthanasia or physician-assisted suicide. This ensures that palliative care clinicians

Box 6.8 Typical Application Requirements for Voluntary Assisted Dying or Euthanasia

• Be suffering a serious and incurable disease or a serious, chronic, and incapacitating condition in the terms established by the Law, certified by the responsible physician.

• Have information available to them on their medical care, alternatives to and possibilities of their request, including access to comprehensive palliative care and dependency care benefits.

• The interested party must request medical assistance in dying twice in writing (or by other means if the person cannot write), generally 10–15 days apart, and expressly explaining that it is not the result of any external pressure. After the first request, the responsible physician of the patient must confirm the diagnosis, prognosis, possible therapies, as well as possible palliative care, ensuring that the patient understands the information provided to them. After that, the patient must confirm their intention.

• Give informed consent prior to receiving assistance to die.

• The patient must have the agreement of their coordinating physician. The latter must request the opinion of another consulting physician with training in the field of the patient's pathologies, who must not belong to the same team as the responsible physician. Afterward, in several countries, there is an evaluation commission that will appoint two experts to evaluate the case (one of them a lawyer). If both agree, the process will move forward. If not, the full commission must decide. Once it has been decided that the request is justified, the responsible physician will be informed, so that they can proceed to apply for euthanasia or assisted suicide. If at any stage the request is rejected, the interested party can appeal to the commission.

sustain hope in the remaining life of each patient and avoid palliative care being deemed futile.

Recording and Communicating

The interdisciplinary team must assure themselves of the preferred language and communication style of the patient and family. Adequate communication skills are required to be able to openly and honestly address and discuss end of life concerns, break bad news, disclose prognosis, and understand hopes, fears, or expectations in the context of social and cultural customs in a developmentally appropriate manner.

When necessary, written information will be provided in a way that the patient and family can read and understand. For whatever scenario, health professionals will ensure proper understanding of the situation, as well as the decisions made to approach the end.

Policies and Protocols

Most healthcare centers and home care teams rely on a protocol to accompany a patient as he or she approaches death.

Most protocols have as objectives:

* To accompany the patient and family throughout the process of dying and final days, providing them with all the necessary care they require, ensuring that this process is as inclusive as possible, and the final act will bestow a *good death*.
* To humanize the process of dying in such a way that professionals' actions address the needs of the patient, who wants to be treated as a person.

Most teams organize a meeting with the family to be able to talk about the subject of dying and define what nearing the end will be like.

Teams and Supervision

Caregiver fatigue and burnout have been described in the literature for some time among professionals who care for patients in situations with great emotional impact (see Chapter 11). In recent decades, various initiatives have been put in place with the aim of caring for the caregiver.

Some teams have implemented mindfulness, yoga, and psychological supervision with the aims of improving well-being and self-care, and of minimizing or even preventing any emotional impact that can often be transferred to professional teams from the constant exposure to, and care for, dying and suffering patients.

Notes

* We use the term "wish to hasten death" (WTHD), attributable to an international study carried out with 24 experts in the field. Due to the lack of precision and consistency in the terminology used in the previous literature, a sufficiently broad expression was sought, and an attempt was made to detail its content. See Balaguer A, Monforte-Royo C, Porta-Sales J, et al. An international consensus definition of the wish to hasten death and its related factors. PLoS One. 2016;11(1):e0146184. doi: 10.1371/journal.pone.0146184. Erratum in: PLoS One. 2018 Apr 26;13(4):e0196754.

References

1. Lau F, Cloutier-Fisher D, Kuziemsky C, Black F, Downing M, Borycki E, et al. A systematic review of prognostic tools for estimating survival time in palliative care. J Palliat Care. 2007;23:93–112.
2. White N, Harries P, Harris AJL, et al. How do palliative care doctors recognise imminently dying patients? A judgement analysis. BMJ Open. 2018;8:e024996.
3. White N, Reid F, Harris A, Harries P, Stone P. A systematic review of predictions of survival in palliative care: How accurate are clinicians and who are the experts? PLoS One. 2016;11(8):e0161407.

4. Steinhauser KE, Clipp EC, McNeilly M, Christakis NA, McIntyre LM, Tulsky JA. In search of a good death: Observations of patients, families, and providers. Ann Intern Med. 2000;132(10):825–832.

5. Steinhauser KE, Christakis NA, Clipp EC, McNeilly M, McIntyre L, Tulsky JA. Factors considered important at the end of life by patients, family, physicians, and other care providers. JAMA. 2000;284(19):2476–2482.

6. Maltoni M, Caraceni A, Brunelli C, et al. Prognostic factors in advanced cancer patients: evidence-based clinical recommendations—a study by the Steering Committee of the European Association for Palliative Care. J Clin Oncol. 2005;23:6240–6248.

7. Cherny N, Fallon N, Kaasa S, Portenoy RK, Currow DC. Oxford Textbook of Palliative Medicine. 6th ed. Oxford: Oxford University Press; 2021.

8. National Consensus Project Steering Committee; Arnold RM, Berger A, et al. Clinical practice guidelines for quality palliative care. Brooklyn, NY: National Consensus Project for Quality Palliative Care; 2004.

9. Monforte-Royo C, Villavicencio Chávez C, Tomás-Sábado J, Balaguer A. The wish to hasten death: A review of clinical studies. Psycho-Oncology. 2011;20:795–804.

10. Balaguer A, Monforte-Royo C, Porta-Sales J, Alonso-Babarro A, Altisent R, Aradilla-Herrero A, et al. An international consensus definition of the wish to hasten death and its related factors. PLoS One. 2016;11(1):e0146184.

11. Monforte-Royo C, Villavicencio Chávez C, Tomás-Sábado J, Mahtani V, Balaguer A. What lies behind the wish to hasten death? A systematic review and meta-ethnography from the perspective of patients. PLoS One. 2012;7(5):e37117.

12. Rodríguez-Prat A, Balaguer A, Booth A, Monforte-Royo C. Understanding patients' experiences of the wish to hasten death: An updated and expanded systematic review and meta-ethnography. BMJ Open. 2017;7(9): e016659.

13. Chochinov HM, Wilson KG, Enns M, et al. Desire for death in the terminally ill. Am J Psychiatry. 1995;152(8):1185–1191.

14. Rosenfeld B, Breitbart W, Galietta M, et al. The schedule of attitudes toward hastened death: Measuring desire for death in terminally ill cancer patients. Cancer. 2000;88(12):2868–2875.

15. Kelly B, Burnett P, Pelusi D, Badger S, Varghese F, Robertson M. Factors associated with the wish to hasten death: A study of patients with terminal illness. Psychol Med. 2003;33(1):75–81.

16. Villavicencio Chávez C, Monforte-Royo C, Tomás-Sábado J, Porta Sales J, Maier M, Balaguer A. Physical and psychological factors and the wish to hasten death in advanced cancer patients. Psycho-Oncology. 2014;23(10):1125–1132.

17. Beck AT, Kovacs M, Weisman AD. Hopelessness and suicidal behaviour. JAMA 1975;234:1146–1149.

18. Guerrero-Torrelles M, Monforte-Royo C, Tomás-Sábado J, Marimon F, Porta-Sales J, Balaguer A. Meaning in life as a mediator between physical impairment and the wish to hasten death in patients with advanced cancer. J Pain Symptom Manage. 2017;54(6):826–834.

19. Monforte-Royo C, Crespo I, Rodríguez A, Marimon F, Porta-Sales J, Balaguer A. The role of perceived dignity, depression, functional impairment and control in the wish to hasten death among advanced cancer patients: A mediation model. Psycho-Oncology. 2018;27(12):2840–2846.

20. Breitbart W, Rosenfeld B, Gibson C, et al. Impact of treatment for depression on desire for hastened death in patients with advanced AIDS. Psychosomatics. 2010;51(2):98–105.

21. Bellido-Pérez M, Monforte-Royo C, Tomás-Sábado J, Porta-Sales J, Balaguer A. Assessment of the wish to hasten death in patients with advanced disease: A systematic review of measurement instruments. Palliat Med. 2017;31(6):510–525.

22. Crespo I, Monforte-Royo C, Balaguer A, et al. Screening for the wish to hasten death in the first palliative care encounter: A proof-of-concept study. J Palliat Med. 2021;24(4):570–573.

23. Zeng YS, Wang C, Ward KE, Hume AL. Complementary and alternative medicine in hospice and palliative care: A systematic review. J Pain Symptom Manage. 2018;56(5):781–794.e4.

24. Candy B, Armstrong M, Flemming K, et al. The effectiveness of aromatherapy, massage and reflexology in people with palliative care needs: A systematic review. Palliat Med. 2020;34(2):179–194.

25. Frerich G, Romotzky V, Galushko M, et al. Communication about the desire to die: Development and evaluation of a first needs-oriented training concept—a pilot study. Palliat Support Care. 2020;18(5):528–536.

26. Breitbart W, Rosenfeld B, Gibson C, et al. Meaning-centered group psychotherapy for patients with advanced cancer: A pilot randomized controlled trial. Psycho-Oncology. 2010;19(1):21–28.

27. Chochinov HM, Hack T, Hassard T, Kristjanson LJ, McClement S, Harlos M. Dignity therapy: a novel psychotherapeutic intervention for patients near the end of life. J Clin Oncol. 2005;23:5520–5525.

28. Griffiths RR, Johnson MW, Carducci MA, et al. Psilocybin produces substantial and sustained decreases in depression and anxiety in patients with life-threatening cancer: A randomized double-blind trial. J Psychopharmacol. 2016;30(12):1181–1197.

29. Ross S, Bossis A, Guss J, et al. Rapid and sustained symptom reduction following psilocybin treatment for anxiety and depression in patients with life-threatening cancer: A randomized controlled trial. J Psychopharmacol. 2016;30(12):1165–1180.

30. Fan W, Yang H, Sun Y, et al. Ketamine rapidly relieves acute suicidal ideation in cancer patients: A randomized controlled clinical trial. Oncotarget. 2017;8(2):2356–2360.

Further Reading

Breitbart W, Rosenfeld B, Pessin H, et al. Depression, hopelessness, and desire for hastened death in terminally ill patients with cancer. JAMA. 2000;284(22):2907–2911. Study of factors related to a desire for hastened death.

Cherny N, Fallon N, Kaasa S, Portenoy RK, Currow DC, Editors. Oxford Textbook of Palliative Medicine. 6th ed. Oxford: Oxford University Press; 2021. Reference textbook for professionals in palliative care.

Monforte-Royo C, Villavicencio Chávez C, Tomás-Sábado J, Balaguer A. The wish to hasten death: A review of clinical studies. Psychooncology. 2011;20:795–804. A broad systematic review that includes 289 studies about the wish to hasten death.

National Consensus Project Steering Committee; Arnold RM, Berger A, et al. Clinical Practice Guidelines for Quality Palliative Care. Brooklyn, NY: National Consensus Project for Quality Palliative Care; 2004. Guideline for quality palliative care.

Chapter 7

Carer, Partner, and Family-Centered Support

Hannah-Rose Mitchell, Allison J. Applebaum, and Talia Zaider

Learning Objectives

After reading this chapter the clinician will be able to:

1. Recognize cancer-related distress and psychosocial challenges in the caregiver, partner, and family extending to the end of life phase.
2. Confidently assess the psychosocial support needs of patients, their caregivers, partners, and family.
3. Provide appropriate supportive care to help alleviate distress.
4. Identify psychosocial referrals for the caregiver, partner, and family.
5. Incorporate relevant ethical, cultural, and professional factors in working with the caregiver, partner, and family in the palliative and end of life setting.

Background Evidence

Cancer is a family problem. Its impact extends beyond the patient to the entire family. As cancer care responsibilities are shifted to the home, the family is increasingly exposed to and involved with the patient's illness, treatment, and transition to palliative care.[1] The impact of cancer on the family is complicated by the growing number of family members and friends tasked with serving as *caregivers* and providing multiple complex care tasks to the patient throughout the care continuum through the end of life phase. These caregivers are often catapulted without warning into simultaneously coping with the experience of illness in the family, while adjusting to the caregiver role and its impact on their routine and identity, and any resulting relational changes with the patient and family.[1,2] It is not just those serving in the caregiver role who are affected by cancer. Cancer poses a major disruption to the entire *family system*, commonly the patient's partner as well as children, parents, and other family members or close friends and nonrelated families of choice. Couples and families are required to balance illness and nonillness priorities, and allocate time and financial resources to meet family members with cancer's illness-related needs, navigate the end of life phase, while managing the ongoing needs and goals of the family.[3]

The responsibilities of caregiving often directly cause distress, in part because caregivers are frequently unprepared for the range of tasks assumed of them. As a result, the majority of caregivers may experience role strain and caregiver burden.[4] The diffuse distress associated with caregiving is linked to immediate and long-term negative health consequences. Around 20% of caregivers report that providing cancer caregiving has made their health worse.[5] Caregivers have excess risk for sleep disturbances, neuroendocrine dysregulation, reduced immune functioning, pain, and excess risk for cardiovascular disease. Cancer caregivers are at risk for overall impaired quality of life and increased morbidities and early mortality.[4]

Factors like the relationship quality between the patient–caregiver/partner dyad and the functioning of the family can predict how individuals and families will cope with cancer.[6] Some families and individuals may be more or less vulnerable to the psychosocial impact of cancer in the family. Caregiving responsibilities may be distributed and shared in supportive and well-functioning families, but those with difficulty functioning may experience more disruption. Relational challenges include role change, communication difficulties, conflict, and anger, navigating boundaries, and intimacy. These can occur at the dyadic level or within the broader family system throughout the care continuum and during the palliative care and end of life phase.

🔍 Key Point

The experience of patients and their partners/family system/caregivers can be interdependent. Coregulation of distress occurs such that the goals, needs, and emotional experiences of patients and family members tend to be highly related.[6]

Cancer presents many unknowns that engender feelings of fear and uncertainty in the patient and family. The concerns associated with the illness itself, in combination with changes in routine, relationships, and family structure, can contribute to high levels of psychological distress. Caregivers, partners, or any family members are at risk for psychiatric symptoms at levels similar to, or higher than, the patient.[4,7]

The impact of cancer on the family will likely persist beyond the patient's death and into the bereavement phase. Family members require support during this transition and efforts to reduce lasting morbidity as a consequence of complicated grief. Challenges in family functioning may predispose family members to negative psychosocial consequences during bereavement, and thus should be identified early. Caregivers may incur increased responsibilities as the patient's death approaches and may experience elevated distress and feelings of relief and guilt entering the bereavement phase (see also Chapter 10 on bereavement care).

🔍 Key Point

Prevention and mitigation of complicated grief can be achieved by improving family functioning and the end of life experience for patients and caregivers.

Thus, clinicians should aim to identify families and caregivers who could benefit from intervention to strengthen family coping and reduce caregiver distress.

In recent years, while the number of studies assessing interventions to reduce distress in caregivers, couples, and families has increased, empirical support for these interventions in palliative care and at the end of life is somewhat limited. Most interventions in advanced cancer delivered to patients and caregivers have used educational methods to improve coping and facilitate communcation and problem-solving, and show some support for improvement in relationship functioning and reduction of caregiver burden.[8] Access and logistical barriers, such as lack of time, present challenges to caregiver and family engagement in psychosocial interventions in pallitative care. However, efforts to engage caregivers and families centrally in routine palliative care delivery have shown efficacy in reducing patient and caregiver distress. [8]

Together the literature suggests that the psychosocial impact of cancer must be recognized as a family problem and understood in terms of interpersonal relationships. The cancer experience involves transitions for those taking on the caregiver role and in the couples' life and family system, which continue through the end of life phase and into bereavement. The shifts in relationships and family dynamics result in consequences on quality of life often beyond what is immediately visible to the oncology providers or even noticed by families themselves. Thus, screening to identify partners, families, and caregivers "at risk" for higher burden and psychological distress is an important priority for all members of the healthcare team, and referral to appropriate psychosocial care is likewise necessary.

Presenting Problems

Key Symptoms and Signs

Clinicians need to be able to recognize presenting psychosocial or relationship problems that cause functional impairment. These problems also serve as predictors of complicated grief and continuing need for bereavement care. Thus, their identification warrants further screening about existing coping skills and preparedness for death. Common key symptoms and signs of impairment due to cancer in the family are shown in Box 7.1 and described in more detail below.

⚲ Caregiving Challenges

- **Burden.** Many families and caregivers experience caregiver burden, a multidimensional response including the emotional, social, and financial impact of caregiving.

Where this occurs, caregivers may present:

- Feelings of dread, especially around caregiving duties
- Difficulty regulating emotions (e.g., uncertainty, guilt, anger, resentment)

Box 7.1 Key Symptoms and Signs for Caregivers and Families

Caregiver Challenges
- Burden
- Role Strain
- Anticipatory Grief

Relational Challenges
- Role Changes
- Communication Difficulty
- Conflict/Anger
- Navigating Boundaries
- Intimacy Concerns

Subclinical/Clinical Psychiatric Symptoms
- Anxiety
- Depression
- Posttraumatic Stress

- Externalized emotions and subsequent conflict
- Insomnia or sleep disturbances
- Unhealthy coping strategies such as substance use or unhealthy eating
- Deferring one's own preventative or follow-up medical care.

These experiences, in combination with prolonged elevated stress levels, render caregivers vulnerable to poor physical health outcomes. Caregiver burden may be exacerbated at the end of life and linked to complicated grief. Caregivers with heightened burden often report feelings of relief and guilt after the patient's death.

- **Role strain.** Juggling multiple roles often involves competing demands on caregiver resources, time, and energy. A cancer diagnosis is usually unexpected, and caregivers are required to perform unfamiliar and time-consuming tasks to provide support to the patient. Such tasks may intensify during the palliative care phase, and as the patient's health status declines and they become frailer. Caregivers experiencing role strain may notice increasing schedule demands and subsequent challenges with time management. The role strain associated with caregiving and the schedule demands have been shown to contribute to persistent emotional distress.

- **Anticipatory grief.** Caregivers may begin to experience the psychological consequences of the care recipient's death while they are still alive. This form of grief is known as anticipatory, or pre-loss, grief. Grieving the loss of the prior quality of life enjoyed before their loved one's cancer and the traumatic distress of facing the life-threatening illness, compounded with anticipation of the patient's death may precipitate the grieving process in caregivers and families (see Chapter 10 on bereavement care).

⚲ Relational Challenges

- **Role changes.** Family members often experience significant disruptions to their usual roles due to a cancer diagnosis and its treatment. As loved ones take on the role of the caregiver, they may experience a loss of mutuality in their relationship with the patient. Adult children of cancer patients sometimes experience a role reversal, as they become responsible for providing care to those who have historically cared for them. The administrative and legal designation of "patient" and "caregiver" or healthcare proxy roles introduces expectations and responsibilities around the patient's care and medical decision-making. When roles are rigidly assumed by family members, this can put strain on a relationship that is unable to adapt when the demands of the illness change (e.g., from a crisis stage to a chronic or remission stage). Caregivers may also serve as "gatekeepers," and perceive that their responsibility is to protect the patient from any stress, which may result in a sense of isolation or burden for the caregiver, and a diminished sense of agency for the patient. Challenges also can arise over distribution of cancer management tasks, such as scheduling appointments, checking medication lists, communicating concerns and advocating to providers, and planning for death. When the patient–caregiver dyad has a history of conflict around control and responsibility, the allocations of care management tasks may also result in friction.

- **Communication difficulty.** Those coping with illness in the family often endorse communication challenges such as withholding fears about prognosis, death, or sense of burden from treatment side-effects. For couples in particular, changes in sexual functioning or physical appearance following treatment may be taboo topics. Oftentimes, discussion of death and dying is limited due to its taboo nature. Discussions around death could involve a range of topics including where to die, funeral planning/the nature of memorial and remembering, and expectations and concerns for bereavement. Couples with poor or limited communication may have fewer opportunities to engage with and support each other effectively, which can lead to further distancing and sense of loss.

- **Conflict/anger.** The chronic strain of illness in the family can deepen long-standing fractures in relationships. Families with poorer functioning and greater conflict to begin with may be more vulnerable to tension under the strain of the illness. Partners and other family members, especially those serving in the caregiver role may express anger and feelings of resentment (e.g., "I didn't sign up for this"). Conflict can also arise when caregivers blame the patient for their diagnosis or progression of illness. This may occur when there has been a history of high-risk health behaviors (e.g., substance use, tobacco, unprotected sex/HPV infection) or when the patient has been nonadherent to treatment or surveillance recommendations. Conflict among the patient's multiple family members or caregivers may arise related to end of life decision-making.

- **Navigating boundaries.** Families of a patient receiving palliative care may find themselves negotiating new boundaries with extended family and others in the wider social support network who are involved in aspects of patient care. Family involvement can take on multiple forms, from active involvement in treatment or end of life decision-making, to contributing professional or personal knowledge that helps the family navigate and interface with providers and healthcare systems. This involvement can elevate the roles of certain individuals over others. The family unit may expand to include broader support. For example, an adult child or an extended relative could swiftly take on a more dominant role in the family that dilutes the cohesiveness of the patient and their partner. Boundary challenges may arise due to individuals moving in or out of their homes to help with other family members. It becomes challenging for family members to maintain their sense of agency and continuity of their relationships, especially couples. For other families, geographic isolation from broader family systems presents an obstacle to obtaining adequate support. Additionally, separated couples sometimes re-engage for support, often with a sense of responsibility but confusion around boundaries and ambivalence about the relationship.

- **Intimacy concerns.** A concern specific to couples and intimate partners during palliative care involves the impact of cancer-related changes in physical appearance and/or sexual functioning. Expectations around engaging in intimacy during the end of life may be quite limited. Couples coping with these concerns can have difficulty acknowledging the loss of physical intimacy. Patients sometimes report body image concerns or fears about attractiveness to their partner. Both partners may endorse complaints about reduced physical affection and physical engagement. These concerns can be compounded by partners' difficulty communicating their level of sexual desire or lack thereof.

⚘ Subclinical/Clinical Psychiatric Symptoms

Cancer has the potential to precipitate elevated levels of *anxiety, depression,* and *posttraumatic stress* (see Chapters 2, 3, and 4), which impair quality of life and functioning, and in some cases meet clinical diagnostic cutoffs. Around the initiation of cancer treatment, anxiety and depression tend to be elevated among caregivers, and these symptoms fluctuate throughout the illness trajectory, with elevations due to adverse illness- or treatment-related events, decline in the patient's health status, and approaching end of life.

The negative emotions that arise following illness in the family are likely to perpetuate mood symptoms. For example, caregivers may suffer from low self-esteem, as they tend to report feelings of ineptitude in providing care. A cancer diagnosis can also be very socially isolating, as family members are forced to prioritize the patient's care over other obligations and activities that help them to feel connected. Feelings of hopelessness are also not uncommon. Family members of a cancer patient also face a great deal of uncertainty and may develop worries and fears about the patient's prognosis, their own involvement in care, and preparedness for the loss of the patient. Fear of disease progression and mortality may underlie or exacerbate anxiety and PTSD symptoms.

The following principles guide the assessment process used to define couple, family, and caregiver concerns, identify the prominent dynamics, and help the patient and unit of care reach agreement about the goals of psychosocial care that may follow this assessment.

- *Identifying the unit of care.* A patient- and family-centered, culturally responsive, and clinically flexible approach should be taken to identify the unit of care. Patients and caregivers should mutually agree to the caregivers' role. The unit of care could include biological relatives or nonbiological friends/relatives or families of choice. When there are multiple people involved in caregiving, and there typically are, providers should be judicious and use the patient's input to determine whom to engage in the care process and how to best engage with them. This can be achieved with an initial assessment of the presenting patient followed by assessment of the caregiver or couple/family together when it appears indicated. Moreover, it is important to assess the capacity of the unit of care to deliver complex care or palliative care to frail patients with advanced and progressive cancer.

- *Relational vs. individual needs.* There must be flexibility in understanding and recognition of individual versus relational needs in the caregiving unit. There should be ongoing assessment to account for changing preferences and family dynamics at different phases of the care journey. As the patient approaches end of life, caregiver roles and preparedness for levels of involvement may become more central concerns. The treatment team must work to balance patient wishes with caregivers' ability and readiness to carry out patient's goals of care. If the patient presents for a psychosocial assessment with family members, clinicians can inquire about the patient's desire to have loved ones join them in the consultation. When there are differences in preferences (e.g., partner desires to join the patient, but the patient wishes to be seen alone), providers can suggest seeing the patient for a portion of the session, with the partner joining for the remainder of the appointment. It can also be useful to consider the referral (i.e., was the couple or family unit referred for assessment). In an initial assessment, problems specific to the caregiver experience, related to the relational dynamics in the couple/family system, or related to individual distress or psychiatric symptoms in the patient or caregiver may all arise and require different treatment approaches involving one or more members of the unit of care.

- *Strengths alongside concerns.* Clinicians should aim to identify the evident individual and interpersonal strengths within the unit of care. Doing so will shift the focus towards healing and potential gains without magnifying deficits. It can facilitate buy-in and self-efficacy in those considering initiating treatment. Of course, challenges and areas of focus should be identified as well to inform treatment. This holistic approach also normalizes psychosocial assessment, which should not be limited to higher needs couples and families. Identifying strengths can contribute to resilience and growth in any individual or family following a cancer diagnosis and lasting into bereavement.

- **Synthesis of findings and goal-setting.** Assessment should ultimately culminate in feedback synthesizing areas of strength and resilience, as well as areas of concern that are useful for the patient and family to consider and address. The clinician, patient, and their unit of care should work to reach agreement about a small number of goals or targets. These will establish an agenda for the family, identify any necessary referrals, and inform a focus for intervention. Discussion of goals for end of life should be facilitated in the couple and family. For example, establishing goals and plans for care at home, for respite for the caregiver, and for place of death, should be encouraged.
- **Timing of assessment.** The optimal approach to assessment is to offer caregivers and families assessment and consultation around the time of entry into palliative care, and then continuously through bereavement. Early assessment of caregivers and families that is integrated into the patient's care is more likely to be construed as preventative and normative. Assessment should be ongoing as multiple novel stressors present throughout the care continuum and as the family becomes closer to facing the patient's death, and individual and family circumstances and resources are also likely to fluctuate. Assessment of the caregivers, partners, and the broader family system should occur even if there is not any evident distress or dysfunction, given the high levels of caregiver and family distress that are often overlooked.
- **History of dealing with loss and death.** Family and caregiver coping resources and strategies, as well as their attitudes and experiences around death should be assessed. Cultural, religious, and spiritual beliefs around death and dying should be considered. The family's historical experiences with death, practices to memorialize lost family members, and the extent to which they feel comfortable discussing death within the family can be predictive of the family's preparedness for the death of the patient.

Case Study: Presentation and Assessment

An 84-year-old white Latino, widowed man with stage IV colon cancer, metastasized to the liver, who was receiving palliative care treatment for cancer pain at the end of life, presented to clinic. He was accompanied by his daughter (caregiver), a 51-year-old white Latina teacher.

In his individual assessment, the patient reported several strengths including a strong social support system, expressing gratitude for his daughter and his son-in-law, with whom he lived. He also reported a good relationship with his 49-year-old son, who was an emergency medicine physician at a large hospital system at the opposite side of the country, who he noted was instrumental in guiding some of his care decisions. He also described being very spiritual and religious, and reported connection with his church community prior to the COVID-19 pandemic, which has hindered his ability to socialize and attend church services in person. Several individual concerns were identified. The patient described feeling like a burden on his daughter and her family. He also endorsed existential distress as he approached the end of life.

The primary caregiver (daughter) was assessed separately and then with the patient per the family's request. She reported burden and limited support from family and friends. She felt responsible for her father's pain management and palliative care, including coordinating treatment and scheduling appointments. She endorsed caregiving as a family "duty," and a cultural value of familism, or prioritizing family. She reported feeling overwhelmed and unprepared and low self-efficacy in caregiving. She reported depression and posttraumatic stress symptoms, including insomnia, anhedonia, guilt, avoiding thinking/talking about her father's cancer, recurring nightmares, and anxiety and agitation, especially when encountering any cancer-related stimuli. She reported fear of her father's death and concern about the potential psychological impact on her entire family upon losing the patriarch.

The patient and his daughter indicated that the cancer had disrupted family dynamics and resulted in some conflict, specifically involving the younger physician brother who lived in a distant state. The daughter described her brother as "inconsistently involved" in her father's care and implied that he lacked understanding of her father's advanced illness. She stated that her brother actively questioned their father's medical providers and treatment decisions, and stated he was interested in identifying a clinical trial for his father at his hospital system but did not follow through. She reported that it was difficult for her to communicate with her brother and share the details of her father's end of life status, which she herself was grappling to accept. She stated that she often requested that her husband communicate with her brother for her, and it was important for her to protect her father from becoming aware of any potential conflict between her and her brother. The caregiver also endorsed concerns about the impact of the family's emotional distress on her adolescent children, who lived with and were close with their dying grandfather.

Investigations for Key Differential Diagnosis

There are a variety of predicaments that ought to be watched for and explored, as outlined in Table 7.1. Parallel approaches to more detailed assessment operate for each predicament.

⚲ Useful Screening Measures

For family members facing caregiver-specific challenges (e.g., overwhelmed with new care tasks, juggling multiple roles and responsibilities):
- **Caregiver Burden:** 29-item Zarit Burden interview[9]
- **Caregiver-Specific Distress:** CancerSupportSource®-Caregiver (CSS-CG): 33-item multidimensional distress screen[10]

For couples and families reporting interpersonal challenges within the family:
- **Relational Functioning:** 12-item Family Relationships Index for relational patterns of communication, conflict resolution and cohesion or teamwork[11]
- **Marital distress:** 7-item Dyadic Adjustment Scale[12]

Table 7.1 Key Differentials and Diagnostic Considerations

⚠ Key Differentials and Diagnostic Considerations	Screening/Intervention
Limited caregiver capacity/substantial care needs requiring additional support (home health aides) or placement outside the family	• Physical and occupational therapy assessments for mobility and safety • Social work assessment
Misunderstanding regarding cancer prognosis and treatment and its gravity among family members	• Family meetings for assessment of understanding and interdisciplinary patient/family education
Undiagnosed psychiatric disorder or drug and alcohol abuse in patient, caregiver, partner, or family member	• Brief distress or substance use (e.g., CAGE assessment) screening • Identification of appropriate referral for individual therapy, medication management
Domestic/intimate partner violence	• Inquiry about present or past experiences of physical, emotional and verbal harm/abuse • Inquiry about whether a partner or family member has interfered with treatment adherence or recovery • WAST (Women's Abuse Screening Tool), HITS (Hurts, Insults, Threatens, Screams) • Notification of social worker and/or primary treatment team when concerns arise • Providing patient with hotline numbers and/or safety planning resources
Additional caregiving needs in the family (e.g., disabled, or ill child, or elderly parent with high care needs)	• Social work assessment • Respite care
Socioeconomic, cultural or language barrier issues, including inability to access necessary patient support at home	• Social work and financial planning assessment • Identification of interpreter services
Specialized support needs of children/adolescents in the family who may be distressed	• Asking patients with minor children whether there are concerns about the support needs of children at home • Identification of appropriate referral
Identification of the family's point person or navigator and the trusted contact on the primary oncology team and assess concerns about communication with care team	• Discussion with healthcare proxy about readiness to serve in this role • Documentation of healthcare proxy contact information

For individual patients, caregivers, and family members, reporting psychological distress:

• **Depression:** 9-item PHQ-9 questionnaire for major depression[13]
• **Anxiety:** 7-item GAD-7 questionnaire for anxiety disorder[14]
• **PTSD:** 20-item PCL-5 for posttraumatic stress disorder[15]

Clinical Management

The following flowchart (see Figure 7.1) outlines potential paths of assessment and treatment of members of the unit of care.

Caregiver Support

Targeted empirically supported interventions, which have proliferated over the past decade, include tools to address the unique psychosocial needs of cancer caregivers. The following are examples of clinical strategies and corresponding evidence-based caregiver-focused psychosocial treatment options. While empirical support for these interventions addressing palliative care/end of life specific needs remains somewhat limited, these interventions are generally considered acceptable when delivered at all stages of the care continuum.

✎ Providing Psychoeducation

Clinicians can provide psychoeducation to caregivers to facilitate in-depth knowledge and fact-based understanding of the experience of family caregiving and the impact of cancer on the family.

- Building a therapeutic alliance, delivering fact-based content, and facilitating self-reflection and adaptive coping are the core techniques of psychoeducation.
- Psychoeducation enhances self-awareness and contextual knowledge in order to empower caregivers to engage in healthy, constructive behaviors that can mitigate distress and improve their quality of life.
- Caregiver psychoeducation may focus on skills in managing patient symptoms, providing home-based care to cancer patients, problem-solving coping, improving communication skills, and accessing social support.[8]

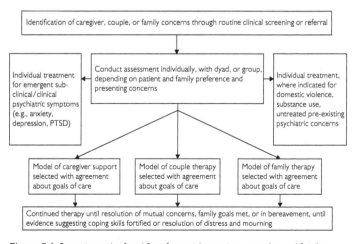

Figure 7.1 Screening and referral flow for at-risk caregivers, couples, and families.

An example of an evidence-based psychoeducational intervention that includes all of these specific components is the ENABLE (Educate, Nurture, Advise, Before Life Ends) Caregiver Intervention, which has been associated with reduced depressive symptoms and burden in caregivers.[16]

Challenging and Changing Cognitions and Behaviors

Strategies grounded in the widely disseminated evidence-based therapy, cognitive-behavioral therapy (CBT), can be implemented in caregivers.[17] CBT focuses on changing caregivers' interpretation of their stressors to subsequently alter their emotional response and behavioral consequences.

- CBT promotes problem-solving skills and has been shown to reduce psychological distress and improve adjustment to caregiving. Of note, caregiver CBT interventions have tended to focus on the acute phase of cancer treatment and not the later phases of treatment or bereavement.[17]
- ⚠ Use of CBT in the oncology and palliative care setting may be limited by the CBT model's emphasis on *illogical* and *irrational* automatic thoughts and beliefs. Reframing beliefs for accuracy may be more challenging when caregivers are coping with patients' ongoing changing needs, guarded prognosis, and impending mortality. Deployment of CBT interventions in the oncology setting should thus be patient/caregiver-centered, sensitive, flexible, and adaptive. Cognitive work in CBT should be focused on addressing "unhelpful" automatic thoughts, rather than identifying and restructuring "illogical" thoughts.

Illogical Automatic Thought: *If we lose hope, our father's death will be our fault.*

Positive Coping Thought: *Losing hope will not change the outcome. As we prepare for his death, we can express love and gratitude for our father.*

Unhelpful Automatic Thought: *If we had encouraged our father to get screened sooner, we could have prevented his cancer progression.*

Positive Coping Thought: *We are doing our best at this time to ensure our father receives the best care and to express our love and gratitude.*

Enhancing Meaning

For many caregivers, addressing existential distress or fostering a sense of meaning, purpose, and growth despite the limitations and challenges of caregiving can be protective against poor psychosocial outcomes. Meaning Centered Psychotherapy for Cancer Caregivers (MCP-C) is a psychotherapeutic approach to target common existential concerns in caregivers of patients with cancer. MCP-C aims to connect or reconnect caregivers with various sources of meaning (i.e., historical, attitudinal, creative, experiential).[18] It involves seven hour-long sessions, each of which includes a didactic portion exploring the sources of meaning (see Table 7.2), and experiential exercise questions that help caregivers to explore how these sources of meaning can

Table 7.2 Sources of Meaning in Caregiving

Source	Content	Caregiver Examples
Historical	Legacy given (past), lived (present), and to give (future)	Past experiences with illness and loss or providing/watching others provide care, family values of care, pride in caregiving, setting examples for future generations
Attitudinal	Choosing how to face limitations associated with caregiving: Reflection on preexisting challenges and modes of facing them (e.g., achievements in the face of adversity, transcending difficult circumstances). Discussion of choosing new responses and taking pride in one's attitude.	The choice to provide care, facing limitations due to caregiving, engaging fully in the relationship with the patient despite its possible ending.
Creative	Engaging in and taking responsibility for one's own life through creative acts.	Participating fully in the caregiving role and taking responsibility via improved self-care, and discussion of existential and neurotic guilt.
Experiential	Connecting with life through love, beauty, and humor.	A tight hug or handhold (to feel/express love toward the patient), finding humor in dark moments, and fostering hope from a sense of belonging to something greater than oneself.

become resources for them. It has been supported as an in-person face-to-face treatment and has been adapted to be delivered over the Internet.[19]

꘎ Facilitating Dyadic Coping

Caregiver interventions can also be dyadic, delivered to the patient–caregiver dyad with the goal to simultaneously address the needs of both patient and caregiver and their relationship. Unlike typical couple therapy (described below), caregiver-specific dyadic interventions are focused on the demands of illness, problem solving, treatment decisions and facilitating support between the patient–caregiver dyad. They aim to improve communication and foster dyadic coping to manage stress. One example of dyadic intervention, with evidence to improve quality of life, self-efficacy, and coping, is the FOCUS Program[20] (see Box 7.2)

Couple and Family Therapy
Therapy aimed to address the relational strains and disruptions in the couple and family associated with cancer may prove beneficial given the potential

> ### Box 7.2 Components of the FOCUS Program
>
> - **F**amily involvement
>   - *Fosters open-communication, teamwork, support*
> - **O**ptimistic attitude
>   - *Addresses outlook*
> - **C**oping effectiveness
>   - *Promotes active, dyadic coping*
> - **U**ncertainty reduction
>   - *Provides psychoeducation about cancer and treatment and promotes acceptance of uncertainty*
> - **S**ymptom management
>   - *Teaches strategies to manage symptom distress*

for relational challenges throughout the cancer trajectory. The following components are commonly included in couple and family therapy.

✎ Increasing Awareness of Cancer Impact and Preparation for Loss of Life on Family

Discussion of the impact of cancer individually and on relationships can be a useful assessment and intervention tool in couple and family therapy. Discussion about cancer-related impact provides opportunity for in-depth reflection on relationship changes, new family dynamics, and how the couple and family members relate to one another historically and in new ways. This approach involves the clinician asking circular questions to highlight the impact of cancer on each other, and facilitate perspective taking, empathy, and attunement. Open discussion of death and dying should be encouraged among the couple and family. Approaching the often-taboo topic of death can be empowering as the couple and family releases any protective or avoidant stance and takes on a more realistic lens that ultimately facilitates important conversation and planning for end of life. Acknowledging death and dying can also allow opportunity for the family members to express appreciation, acknowledge the transition, and say goodbye to the family member.

✎ Strengthening Communication Skills

Clinicians can aim to strengthen communication, first by observing couple and family communication patterns by prompting discussion of topics of concern. Clinicians should take note of any hesitancy or cautiousness in individual's expression of their thoughts and feelings. Patterns involving criticism, defensiveness, interruption, and withdrawal should also be observed and reflected. Guardedness should be normalized as a common response to cancer that can affect communication. Partners or family members may experience concerns about burdening each other with their distress, and clinicians should encourage discussion of these beliefs, the process of shared coping, and to assess any pressure about the need to reassure or problem-solve in response to emotional disclosures. Clinicians should facilitate reflection on how to optimize disclosure of negative feelings (e.g., grief, fear). Setting communication ground rules may be especially important for conflict-prone couples and families. Communication around end of life issues should be facilitated. Couples may also want to establish strategies for communicating with other members of the family about the death of the patient, such as children.

⚓ Redefining Intimacy

Couples coping with profound changes in physical functioning due to cancer should be supported in re-examining sources of intimacy in their relationship. Clinicians should aim to normalize and facilitate dialogue about changes in sexual functioning and any accompanying feelings of loss and shame, and address concerns about frailty. The clinician should convey that sexuality and intimacy are important at every stage of life, including end of life. The value of physical contact during the end of life transition should be explored. Increased dialogue can reduce any negative assumptions the partners develop about each other. Couples should be encouraged to broaden their understanding of what is considered intimacy in both emotional and physical domains. Partners should be encouraged to express the range of gestures of intimacy they appreciate most. It can be useful for couples to engage in a more proactive intentional approach to intimacy. Because this approach may seem unnatural or forced to the couple, clinicians should supportively encourage the couple to consider it, and offer suggestions such as practicing sensate focus or planning date nights and rituals. Clinicians should account for sexual expression as part of end of life care planning, and ensure privacy for the individuals and couples, and respect and acknowledge couples' desire for privacy. When physical expressions of intimacy are no longer preferred or realistic, couples may experience tremendous emotional intimacy as they support one another. Clinicians can help cultivate the couples' experience of connection by encouraging each partner to communicate authentically and openly and by ensuring responsiveness to such disclosure.

⚓ Strengthening Resilience

Improving the quality of family relationships can mitigate individual family member's distress throughout the cancer trajectory. Family Focused Grief Therapy (FFGT) is an evidence-based therapy, which targets families coping with advanced cancer to strengthen relationships prior to the loss of the patient. FFGT is a time-limited, manualized intervention offered to families with concerns about functioning, identified as "at risk," and begins during palliative care and continues into bereavement. The continuity of FFGT after the patient's death is a unique feature of this treatment, which prioritizes the family members and can improve adjustment during bereavement. FFGT begins with an assessment phase intended to evaluate **communication, cohesiveness,** and **conflict**. Intervention sessions, held every three to four weeks in the inpatient setting or the family's home, review salient concerns, emphasize family strengths, and facilitate discussion around coping and grief. Clinicians use prompts to discuss family communication, cohesiveness, and conflict, and progress in these areas is discussed. These three areas continue to be discussed after the patient's death.

Individual Referral for Clinically Significant Psychiatric Symptoms

Assessment of caregivers, partners, and families should aim to identify those who endorse levels of anxiety, depression, and posttraumatic stress meeting clinical significance. Some family members will present with preexisting psychiatric conditions, and a cancer diagnosis only serves to enhance vulnerability and exacerbate psychological symptoms.

🔍 Key Point

For some patients and caregivers, standard evidence-based psychological treatments like CBT or (ACT) may be warranted to address anxiety and depression symptoms.

Trauma-focused CBT, prolonged exposure, or cognitive processing therapy may be warranted for those presenting with clinically significant PTSD. Insomnia is also common in families coping with cancer, and while symptoms of insomnia may subside by reducing caregiver burden, addressing diffuse distress, and improving relationship functioning, CBT for insomnia (CBT-I) may be of benefit to certain individuals, especially those with history of insomnia prior to the patient's cancer diagnosis. Individual treatment can be accompanied with referral to psychiatry services and psychopharmacological interventions as warranted.

Case Study: Clinical Management

In approaching the final year of his life, the patient identified goals for individual therapy of reducing existential suffering and establishing a plan for death while improving cohesion in his family. This was approached by the patient's individual participation in meaning-centered psychotherapy, and inclusion of his family members at the center of his palliative care. Family meetings were scheduled including the physician son, who participated via telehealth. The goal was to facilitate communication about the patient's prognosis and declining health status, enhance open communication around death and dying, amplify the patient's desires in planning his death, and allow his daughter and son to express their feelings of appreciation for their father.

In parallel, the caregiver daughter engaged in individual caregiver supportive psychotherapy, which aimed to reduce the burden associated with the caregiver experience and subsequent role changes, and to mitigate depression and posttraumatic stress symptoms. Specifically, psychoeducation was employed to normalize the experience of caregiver distress and impart the caregiver with skills for coping with the burden of providing home-based care. As caregiver self-efficacy in caregiving increased, CBT addressed maladaptive cognitions about the caregiving experience, her feelings of guilt, while acknowledging the inherent normative distress. Her cultural values of providing care to the family were recognized and explored. Finally, the caregiver was encouraged to approach stimuli associated with her father's illness through exposure to reduce avoidance symptoms. She reported changes in her beliefs about her responsibility in the patient's medical status and reduced self-blame. She also started to notice improvements in mood. Exposures were effective in helping the caregiver to habituate to distressing reminders of cancer. She reported minor improvements in sleep and was eventually referred for CBT for insomnia to address existing sleep patterns contributing to persistent insomnia.

Professional Issues and Service Implementation

Recording and Communicating Challenges

- Unmet informational needs (e.g., information on diagnosis/prognosis, treatment plan, medication/interventions) should be identified and providers should aim to address them via patient and family education, ideally in the setting of family meetings.
- Individuals at risk for prolonged grief should be identified for bereavement consultation.
- A summary of the family dynamic should be documented for the care team, and should delineate the roles of the family unit of care including relevant healthcare providers.

Common Ethical Dilemmas

- ⚠ Family members or other individuals, not identified by patients as part of their unit of care, may want access to patient medical information or to present psychosocial concerns to the clinical team, **but patients must consent to family involvement**.
- Clinicians must take a neutral stance to preempt being drawn into an alliance with either the patient or one member of the unit of care that could limit trust and responsiveness of the other.
- Competing needs and demands of different family members may arise during treatment of the unit of care, which will require triaging concerns and making additional referrals if necessary. Clinicians must ensure other providers are able to meet the demands of the family members referred out.

Legal Responsibilities

- Clinicians should encourage patients and families to put affairs in order (e.g., care needs of children or other family, healthcare directives, power of attorney, and wills) early in the cancer care continuum.

- Clinicians may help negotiate responsibilities of surrogate decision-maker, or families restricted in their ability to safely provide the patient with care to facilitate the death they want (e.g., dying at home).
- Clinicians are required to refer for caregiver, couple, or family therapy, whenever family members require support or issues present at the dyadic or family level.
- Clinicians must be aware of laws regarding living wills and advance directives, and the extent to which the clinical team must review them, which may vary by region and country.
- Clinicians must be aware of laws regarding medically assisted dying, and the roles and responsibilities of family members, which may vary by region and county.

Policies for Clinical Services

- Caregivers, partners, and families should be a central focus of clinical care per the International Association of Hospice and Palliative Care.
- Oncology consultations should invite and encourage partners or relatives attending with patients, including all members of the unit of care in the process, to highlight their expectation for family-centered care. Adaptive use of telehealth should be implemented to involve family members unable to be physically present during consultations.
- Caregiver and family distress screening should be routine and ongoing.
- When children are involved, clinicians must immediately recognize the principle of family-centered care informing clinical practice.
- Caregivers should be identified, and their contact information documented in the patient's (and when possible, their own) chart via a formal process, and they should be provided education in advance of discharge planning. This is exemplified in the United States by the Caregiver Advise Record Enable (CARE) act, legislation enacted to support caregivers in providing unpaid medical care at home, which was signed into law in 40 US states as of 2020.

Teams and Supervision Strategies

- A multidisciplinary team allows opportunity for different perspectives, expertise, and training experiences to holistically address patient and family needs. The team should take a family-centered approach.
- Supervision and consultation should be available to less experienced clinicians in couple and family clinics at comprehensive cancer centers operating a couple and family clinic. Cotherapy models can be used to develop experience within the team and train less experienced clinicians in providing care to caregivers, couples, and families.
- Supervision of couple and family therapists providing psycho-oncology care can use a peer-group model to amplify diverse perspectives to develop hypotheses and strategies about optimal ways to support the patient and family.

References

1. Kent EE, Mollica MA, Buckenmaier S, Wilder Smith A. The characteristics of informal cancer caregivers in the United States. Sem Oncol Nursing. 2019;35(4):328–332. https://doi.org/10.1016/j.soncn.2019.06.002.

2. Girgis A, Lambert S, Johnson C, Waller A, Currow D. Physical, psychosocial, relationship, and economic burden of caring for people with cancer: A review. J Oncol Pract. 2013;9(4):197–202. https://doi.org/10.1200/JOP.2012.000690.

3. Zaider T, Steinglass P. Medical family therapy in oncology. In Clinical Methods in Medical Family Therapy. New York: Springer; 2018. Pages 207–230.

4. Bevans M, Sternberg EM. Caregiving burden, stress, and health effects among family caregivers of adult cancer patients. JAMA. 2012;307(4):398–403. https://doi.org/10.1001/jama.2012.29

5. Hunt, GG, Longacre, M, Kent, EE, Weber-Raley, L. Cancer Caregiving in the U.S.: An Intense, Episodic, and Challenging Care Experience. Washington, DC: National Alliance for Caregiving; 2016.

6. Teixeira RJ, Applebaum AJ, Bhatia S, Brandão T. The impact of coping strategies of cancer caregivers on psychophysiological outcomes: An integrative review. Psychol Res Behav Manage. 2018;11:207–215. https://doi.org/10.2147/PRBM.S164946.

7. Streck BP, Wardell DW, LoBiondo-Wood G, Beauchamp JES. Interdependence of physical and psychological morbidity among patients with cancer and family caregivers: Review of the literature. Psycho-Oncology. 2020;29(6):974–989. https://doi.org/10.1002/pon.5382.

8. Badr H, Krebs P. A systematic review and meta-analysis of psychosocial interventions for couples coping with cancer. Psycho-Oncology. 2013;22(8):1688–1704.

9. Zarit SH, Reever KE, Bach-Peterson J. Relatives of the impaired elderly: Correlates of feelings of burden. Gerontologist. 1980;20(6):649–655. https://doi.org/10.1093/geront/20.6.649.

10. Buzaglo J, Zaleta AK, McManus S, Golant M, Miller MF. CancerSupportSource®: Validation of a revised multi-dimensional distress screening program for cancer patients and survivors. Support Care Cancer 2020;28:55–64.

11. Moos RH, Moos BS. Family Environment Scale Manual. Stanford, CA: Consulting Psychologists Press, 1981.

12. Hunsley J, Pinsent C, Lefebvre M, James-Tanner S, Vito D. Construct validity of the short forms of the Dyadic Adjustment Scale. Family Relations. 1995;231–237.

13. Kroenke K, Spitzer RL, Williams JB. The PHQ-9: Validity of a brief depression severity measure. J Gen Int Med. 2001;16(9):606–613. https://doi.org/10.1046/j.1525-1497.2001.016009606.x.

14. Spitzer RL, Kroenke K, Williams JB, Lowe B. A brief measure for assessing generalized anxiety disorder: The GAD-7. Arch Intern Med. 2006;166:1092. https://doi:10.1001/archinte.166.10.1092.

15. Weathers FW, Litz BT, Keane TM, Palmieri PA, Marx BP, Schnurr PP. The PTSD Checklist for DSM-5 (PCL-5). 2013. Scale available from the National Center for PTSD at www.ptsd.va.gov.

16. Dionne-Odom J, Bakitas M, Ferrell B. Psychoeducational interventions for cancer family caregivers. In Applebaum A, Editor. Cancer Caregivers. New York: Oxford University Press; 2019.

17. O'Toole MS, Zachariae R, Renna ME, Mennin DS, Applebaum A. Cognitive behavioral therapies for informal caregivers of patients with cancer and cancer survivors: A systematic review and meta-analysis. Psycho-Oncology. 2017;26(4):428–437. https://doi.org/10.1002/pon.4144.

18. Applebaum AJ, Kulikowski JR, Breitbart W. Meaning-centered psychotherapy for cancer caregivers (MCP-C): Rationale and overview. Pall Support Care. 2015;13(6):1631. https://doi.org/10.1017/S1478951515000450.

19. Applebaum A, Buda K, Schofield E, et al. Exploring the cancer caregiver's journey through web-based meaning-centered psychotherapy. Psycho-Oncology. 2018;27(3):847–856. https://doi.org/10.1002/pon.4583.

20. Titler MG, Visovatti MA, Shuman C, et al. Effectiveness of implementing a dyadic psychoeducational intervention for cancer patients and family caregivers. Support Care Cancer. 2017;25(11):3395–3406. https://doi.org/10.1007/s00520-017-3758-9.

Further Reading

Applebaum AJ, Editor. Cancer Caregivers. New York: Oxford University Press; 2019. Comprehensive multiauthor text describing experiences of cancer caregivers, psychosocial interventions, and policy, legal, and ethical considerations.

Treanor CJ, Santin O, Prue G, et al. Psychosocial interventions for informal caregivers of people living with cancer. Cochrane Database of Systematic Reviews. 2019(6). https://doi.org/10.1002/14651858.CD009912.pub2. Systematic review detailing evidence-based caregiver-specific psychosocial interventions.

Zaider T, Steinglass P. Medical family therapy in oncology. In Mendenhall T, Lamson A, Hodgson J, Baird M, Editors. Clinical Methods in Medical Family Therapy. New York: Springer; 2018. Pages 207–230. A clinically oriented chapter describing techniques and strategies for family care in oncology.

Zaider TI, Kissane DW. Psychosocial interventions for couples and families coping with cancer. In Breitbart WS, Butow P, Jacobsen PB, Lam WT, Lazenby M, Loscalzo MJ, Editors. Psycho-Oncology. 4th ed. Oxford: Oxford University Press; 2021. Pages 481–488. A comprehensive psycho-oncology textbook chapter describing systemic care provision.

Chapter 8

Care of Dependent Children When a Parent Is Dying of Cancer

Jane Turner and Melissa Henry

Learning Objectives

After reading this chapter the clinician will be able to:

1. Describe the impact of parental cancer and death on children based on their developmental stage.
2. List the strategies which have been demonstrated to improve outcomes for children affected by parental cancer.
3. List factors which increase vulnerability of children and families coping with parental cancer and strategies to respond.
4. Reflect on the range of ethical, cultural, and legal/professional issues that may arise in their clinical care of parents with advanced cancer who have dependent children.

Background Evidence

Parents with advanced cancer who have dependent children must negotiate complex treatment decisions while attempting to maintain family function against a background of disease burden, treatment side-effects, and often financial strain related to cost of treatment and/or inability to work.

There is conflicting evidence about the impact of parental illness on child or adolescent quality of life and adjustment. Adolescents generally show a high level of symptoms, attributed to their developmental stage where issues prevail around identity, independence from parental figures, and social relations with peers.[1] Risky behaviors such as alcohol/substance use are a common expression of adolescent conflict, but these are not necessarily greatly increased when a parent is ill.[2]

Across all age/developmental stages premorbid temperament seems an important predictor of internalizing and externalizing behaviors, with shyness predicting internalizing and poor control/high frustration predicting externalizing problems.[1,3] The response of parents to these behaviors will in turn affect child adjustment and the development of sustained problematic behaviors appears to predict long-term functioning.[1,3] The time around communication of serious news is found to be particularly distressing.[1,3] With time, uncertainty and helplessness in children decreases while loneliness and positive emotions remain stable. Central to favorable outcomes is the presence of strong support networks and recognition of the major impact of changes in social circumstances and peer relationships.[4]

Children of parents with cancer need information about their parent's condition that is appropriate to their developmental stage. Typically, this information will need to be adapted over time. Children also need to be able to express their feelings and concerns about the parent's condition.[5] Structured interventions are reported to have some benefit for children of parents facing cancer in terms of family functioning, depressed mood, parenting skills, and child behavior problems.[6]

Talking with Children about Illness and Death

Children have different temperaments and family dynamics. Social and cultural factors affect adjustment as well as the disease burden and emotional response of the parent.

Developmental Considerations

It is helpful to consider childhood developmental stages in order to assist parents to identify and respond to their child's needs and be able to talk about illness and death.

- Young children—up to about 8 years of age:
  Children in this group have limited ability to understand abstract concepts. They are tied to the here and now and generally lack the verbal skills to describe their concerns. Distress is typically communicated through behavior. They often believe in magic, which is promoted in most cultures. For example, a child who has a birthday may be given a cake and told to make a wish as they blow out the candles. Thus, children often believe that their thoughts and actions can influence outcomes. They do not necessarily see events as happening by chance or bad luck and may blame themselves for adversity, for example, thinking that their parent's illness is because they failed to perform a chore requested of them. Children in this age group typically have limited ability to see the world through the eyes of another. They can be egocentric, and anxiety is often prominent "just below the surface." One of the most common fears of children in this age group is of abandonment and because of their magical thinking they may speculate: "*If Daddy could get sick and not look after me then Mommy could get sick too and there would be no-one to look after me.*" This anxiety can then be expressed in behaviors such as clinging or even being naughty.

- From about 8 to 12 years:
  Children are developing greater ability to talk about their concerns, however, play and physical activity remain important ways of dealing with stress. Belonging and fitting in with peers becomes important so having a

parent with no hair, a walking aid, or wearing a pressure garment can be stigmatizing. Practical disruptions to sporting or other activities because of parental illness can be especially distressing.

- Adolescents, from 12–15 (early) to 15–19 (late) years:

  Adolescents are developing capacity for abstract thought, but this can fluctuate. A 13-year-old who can perform complicated algebra may not have the emotional tools to reflect on pending parental death, the aftermath, and how they might cope. The burden of parental cancer can compound the challenges of negotiating identity, personal, social, and vocational roles. Parental assumptions that adolescent children will "step up" and take on increased domestic responsibility can be a twofold stressor—if the adolescent feels that tasks have been imposed on them without discussion it may erode their sense of autonomy, and the additional roles may reduce opportunities for interaction with friends and social activities which otherwise could positively affect coping.

  For those in later adolescence, the tension of individuation from family to pursue career or occupation and forging of romantic relationships can be stressful. They may feel pressure to remain in the previous family roles and experience guilt about embarking on more adult roles.

Talking about Death

A full grasp of the concept of death means recognition that death affects all living things, it is irreversible and the person who has died has no ongoing functional ability. Children comprehend death as a changed state by about 3 years of age. Before this, although there is no concept of death, infants and toddlers demonstrate awareness of separation from a parental figure and changed routines. Children under 3 years have been known to demonstrate behaviors indicating grief for the loss of a parent.

By about 5 or 6 years of age children come to grasp that death is universal and soon after this to appreciate the things that can cause death. Concepts of death are often acquired through nature and the life cycle, such as when they observe the death of animals or insects. Personal mortality is typically understood at around ages 8 or 9. Parental illness can then stimulate fears around one's own mortality. Nevertheless, there could still be the notion of the cancer as being caused by self, contagious, or bargaining to somehow prevent the death of the parent (e.g., acting as an ideal child to save the parent). The concepts of irreversibility, universality, and nonfunctionality are acquired at around 10 years of age.

Discussion about death thus needs to consider the developmental stage of the child. For very young children explanations must be repeated and accompanied by statements that the death is not the child's fault, that despite the death of the parent they are safe and will always be cared for. The surviving parent may find it intensely distressing to be confronted by a young child who asks repeatedly: "*When is Daddy coming home?*" and will need support to continue these discussions.

An adolescent typically has an accurate concept of death akin to what is found in adults. It is still always important to check their understanding of the cancer following explanations given about it.

Presenting Problems

Key Symptoms and Signs

Children can present with both internalizing and externalizing behaviors.

Internalizing Behaviors

This refers to the inward directing of emotions and feelings. It can include withdrawal from normal activities and relationships, the development of physical symptoms, and depressed and anxious mood. Common physical symptoms are stomach pain, breathing problems, headache, decreased appetite and energy, and problems with sleep. Younger children may demonstrate separation anxiety, a fear of strangers, become clingy, latch on to a security blanket or toy, and be afraid of being left alone. They may become unusually silent, with some even presenting with selective mutism. Young children may revert to previous behaviors of sucking their thumb, talking like a baby, and wetting their beds. They may manifest picky eating or lose their appetite.

Adolescent children may become depressed, however this is not always openly expressed as sadness. Withdrawal from normal social activities, deterioration in school performance, and changes in sleep can represent depression. Anger and irritability and complaints of boredom and wanting to spend the day in bed are also suggestive of depression in adolescents.

Paradoxically, internalizing behaviors may not be seen by parents as markers of distress. The child who is quiet and withdrawn demands less immediate attention of the parent who is ill, and there is potential for their needs to be downplayed or overlooked.

Externalizing Behaviors

This refers to the outward directing of emotions such as in aggression or delinquency. Children can throw tantrums and experience disrupted sleep accompanied by nightmares. These changes can be especially pronounced when the family experiences disruptions in routines and parental roles, such as the parent requiring hospitalization or needing to travel away from home for treatment. Parents need to keep in mind that behavioral disturbance can reflect underlying emotions about the illness and find a way to explore these concerns in a gentle caring way, while setting limits as appropriate.

Investigations for Key Differential Diagnosis

Just as no two people with cancer have an identical disease trajectory, no two children react the same way to parental cancer and death. Bereavement in childhood has been implicated as a risk factor for the development of depression and anxiety in adulthood. However, a focus on disorder fails to consider the more subtle but pervasive changes in thinking and worldview and perhaps sense of optimism about the future. The experience of childhood bereavement may affect lifestyle choices and relationships well into adulthood. Grief is not linear, and throughout adult life there may be painful reminders of loss, particularly at times of major milestones such as graduation, marriage, and birth of children, although the distress does not necessarily constitute disorder.

The following describes some of the factors that may affect outcomes for children. Awareness of these issues is important and early intervention may be required, often involving a range of health professionals.

Preexisting Impairments in Parental and Family Emotional Well-Being
It is obvious that the physical condition of the parent who is ill, including inability to perform normal domestic roles, will affect children. There is strong evidence that the psychological state of the parent who is ill and of family functioning have a direct impact on children facing parental illness. Mental illness in either parent can affect the functioning of the family, which in turn can impact children's adjustment. Effects on communication, affective involvement, and family cohesion can be particularly disruptive, especially when a distressed parent frequently expresses intense negative emotions.

For example:

- A parent who is anxious may frequently talk about their symptoms and express fear about a range of issues leading to a "contagion" of family distress.
- A parent who is anxious may be overprotective and limit the child's engagement in normal activities, which would otherwise help the child to adjust.
- A parent who is depressed may be emotionally unavailable and have limited ability to comfort and respond sensitively to their child's distress.
- Children who feel adrift within the family may demonstrate internalizing or externalizing behaviors as described above.
- A parent who is depressed or anxious may fail to recognize the distress of their child, so health professionals need to recognize that identification and treatment of mental illness in the parent is critical not only for the parent, but also for the wellbeing of children and the family.

Notably, some studies have found that overall family function may even be better in the context of parental illness, due to strengthened relationships, a less controlling family environment, a higher level of organization, and a lower level of family conflicts. This is in line with posttraumatic growth, whereby resilience and meaning making is strengthened in the face of adversity.

Families Facing Adversity
Coping with advanced cancer is even more challenging when a family is already facing hardship such as poverty, parental substance abuse, and family violence. Emerging evidence from the field of epigenetics points to long-term adverse outcomes for children who have been exposed to such adversity. Potential outcomes include lifelong hyperresponsivity to stress, which is compounded by reduced capacity to self-soothe and regulate unpleasant affects leading to an increased risk for maladaptive behaviors and poor lifestyle choices. These risk factors may be evident when taking a social history early in the disease course, however the cost of healthcare, loss of employment, and development of depression may occur because of illness and death, leading to increased risk.

Children of Single Parents and Blended Families

Children of single parents may face uncertainty about their future depending on family support. Children may be cared for by several adults, not all of whom are biologically related (for example a child may live with their mother and her new partner and still have contact with their biological father). Family case conferences involving social workers and members of the oncology team should be offered early after the diagnosis of advanced disease so that the complex issues about future care of children can be discussed, and decisions reached in a timely manner.

🔍 Key Point

This involves a series of sensitive discussions rather than a single discrete conversation. It may take several consultations to establish rapport, gain insights into complex family relationships, and develop an understanding of practical factors affecting decision-making.

Children with Developmental Delays or Other Health Problems

A range of neurodevelopmental and other health conditions increase vulnerability. One relatively common example is autism spectrum disorder (ASD), a neurodevelopmental condition associated with deficits in social communication and interactions across multiple contexts. There is a strong genetic predisposition, and it is not rare for parents to have two children with ASD. In most cases of parental cancer, the parents will be aware of the diagnosis of ASD in an affected child. Identification of existing supports and intervention programs will need to be strengthened if a parent has advanced cancer and specialist advice sought about optimal communication of the diagnosis with affected children. The surviving parent of a child with preexisting health problems is vulnerable to isolation and depression, so early involvement of relevant community-based and professional services is critical. School counseling may be a helpful support for the child with developmental delays or health problems.

Adolescent Children

Adolescents are vulnerable because of the risk of externalizing behaviors (for example drug and alcohol use and unprotected sex) which can lead to long-lasting irreversible consequences. Adolescents commonly present with higher levels of anxiety and depression than younger children. As well as grief about the anticipated loss of their parent, adolescents may become more distant or close, act angrily, and be worried about not being able to spend time with friends. Adolescents may worry about their own genetic risk for cancer. Imposition of unilateral rules to accommodate the changed domestic circumstances increases distress, and adolescent daughters appear to be especially vulnerable if they feel they are pushed into parenting younger siblings and assuming increased domestic roles that erode their ability to maintain supportive social relationships. Females are twice as likely to develop depression as males, and this sex difference emerges in early adolescence.

While adolescents have capacity for abstract thought and can conceptualize at some level a future life without their parent, they may have limited capacity for emotional regulation. Outbursts of rage amounting to verbal attacks such as: *"You're ruining my life. Why don't you just die and get on with it"* are not rare. Parents benefit from support and guidance to develop strategies to respond rather than retaliating. A parent who can acknowledge this rebuke and respond: *"Yes, everything is hard, and you don't deserve this. None of us do. I wish you didn't have to go through this"* can "buy time" for the adolescent to calm down and be able to talk about how their distress can be mitigated. Anger and irritability may also be markers of depression in adolescents, who may benefit from offer of some individual counseling, although this needs to be negotiated respectfully.

Case Study 1

Janice was a 34-year-old woman who had metastatic colorectal cancer. She had two children, Jock aged 6 years and Tina aged 4 years. The children had different fathers, and Janice was estranged from both. Janice had resisted any referral to social work or counseling, insisting that she didn't want people telling her what to do. She had a history of drug abuse and had a tense relationship with her parents. As Janice's disease progressed, she was reluctant to consider what would happen to the children but eventually said that her parents would take care of them. Janice's mother presented to the clinic some weeks after Janice's death and said that she wanted to place Jock in an institution as he was "totally out of control." He was abusive to his grandparents and had repeatedly defecated in their bed.

The consultation-liaison psychiatry service was called and met with Janice's mother, who was exhausted. She felt resentful that there had been no outreach or discussion from the clinic and that the care of the children was "dumped on us." Detailed history-taking suggested that Jock in fact had symptoms suggestive of attention deficit hyperactivity disorder (ADHD). After treatment from a specialist child psychiatrist, introduction of medication, and provision of psychoeducation and parenting guidance his behavior dramatically improved and his grandparents were accepting of caring for him in the longer term.

🔍 Key Point

Don't assume that adequate support has been provided for potential caregivers of children after parental death. Early discussion and support may mitigate against failed care arrangements.

Clinical Management

Education and Support for Parents

Parents instinctively desire to protect their children from hurt and distress. A common response of a parent facing life-limiting illness is to avoid open discussion with their children because they "don't want to upset them." The fear that their ultimate death will irreparably damage their children increases distress and compounds the risk of avoidance. Unfortunately, health professionals may mirror parental avoidance. Serious illness in a person with dependent children can arouse personal feelings of sadness and grief in health professionals who may identify with the person and reflect on their own family. They may also often feel that they lack the knowledge and skills to assist parents.

Open communication generally leads to better coping and lessened psychological distress, whereas avoiding communication can lead to poorer mental health and externalizing behaviors. Communication can help support children's coping and address misconceptions. It can help put into words what would otherwise be expressed physically or behaviorally. For example, a child who develops stomach aches when told her mother needed more chemotherapy can be supported to talk about the issues ("*I'm afraid of my mother getting chemotherapy because this means she won't be able to prepare us supper and drive me to my ballet classes.*"). Engaging parents in discussions which promote optimism about their ability to help their children is vital. This occurs in a series of conversations over time. Parents need encouragement to listen and respond to the needs of each child, bearing in mind their individual differences. Confidence can be built by statements like: "*You know your own child best. Let's talk about how this information can fit with what you feel your child needs.*"

⚲ Key Messages

Information and support can be provided in association with routine clinic attendance by a suitably knowledgeable nurse or social worker. The information that follows will not necessarily be given in one consultation, and ideally once rapport is established with the parent/s more challenging issues can be raised. Core information should include:

• Discussion about developmental stages and understanding of illness, tailored to the ages of the child/ren including concepts such as magical thinking and understanding that young children express distress in behavioral terms;

• Explanation that keeping secrets increases children's distress as they sense that something is wrong but feel that they can't talk about their concerns or ask questions;

• The importance of choosing a time and place to communicate serious news based on conditions parents believe will facilitate discussion, avoiding bedtime as it could disrupt sleep;

Box 8.1 Key Messages for Parents

At the outset there are two key messages to convey to parents:

1. Your child will not inevitably be damaged by your illness. It is more about how it is handled than the illness per se. You have it within your power to make this less difficult for your child.

2. As a parent, one of the greatest gifts you can give your child is to bear your own pain and grief and allow your child to talk openly about even scary and awful things. The truth is hard. Secrets are worse.

- In families comprising more than one child, parents may want to communicate with each child individually to ensure communication is age appropriate (especially if the children's ages are very different or it is anticipated they will cope very differently). If so, these meetings should be conducted close to each other (same day) to avoid children feeling they have been left out;
- Young children in particular are fearful of abandonment and need reassurance that they will be safe and looked after "no matter what";
- Children need to be reassured that the cancer is not their fault;
- Routine is very soothing especially for young children. Although maintaining rules can be challenging, abandoning previous discipline increases anxiety and can lead to behavior disturbance and cascading problems at school and with friends;
- Children and adolescents may become concerned about burdening their parents and be reluctant to ask for help or bring friends home for playdates. They should be encouraged to keep an active and fulfilled life and supported in doing so;
- Children may be affected by comments of other children at school. These comments (typically ill-informed) can be spiteful and distressing. Parents should encourage their child/ren to tell them what others say at school so that they can correct misinformation;
- Although there may be a strong desire for privacy, in general letting the school know about parental illness is helpful. Teachers who are aware of the situation at home can discretely monitor the child's behavior and interactions with other children and offer support if needed;
- Communication needs to be age-appropriate, timely, and empathic. The parent needs to give specific, present-focused, and simple straightforward information. Being honest while maintaining hope is key;
- Information is ideally given in stages. Particularly for younger children, their ability to comprehend that something may happen many months into the future is difficult to grasp;
- Communication needs to strike a balance between talking about the impact of the parent's cancer on the children and engaging in normal regular talk and activities.

Box 8.2 Principles for Communicating with Children

- Discussions should be child-centered and aligned with the child's developmental stage
- There is not necessarily a "right" time for discussion.
- Discussions will evolve over time.
- Misperceptions and fear need to be addressed—the cancer is not the child's fault.
- It is OK to talk about scary things. It is OK to be upset.

⚲ Key Message

Instilling Hope in Parents

It cannot be overstated how important it is for parents who are struggling with guilt, fear, and recriminations about the impact of their cancer on their children to be given information that it is *not* inevitable that their child will be damaged, and to instill a sense of optimism about their capacity to help their child to cope and even flourish. Parents need to know that research has identified factors associated with better outcomes even in children facing what seem like overwhelming odds, and encouragement to work on factors they can influence. It is important to introduce these concepts early in the disease trajectory for those with advanced disease. Later, when a parent's health is deteriorating in the terminal phase, the focus is appropriately on decisions about place of care and symptom control and parents may have little emotional or physical capacity to consider these issues.

Better outcomes for children facing adversity are associated with:

* Having a good relationship with at least one adult who shows positive regard and openness to hearing about the child's worries and concerns. Strengthening relationships with the surviving parent and extended family or even a health professional known to the child can help;
* Being seen and valued for who they are;
* Having the chance to achieve mastery—even small skills like skipping and throwing a ball matter for young children. Success in one area can spill over into willingness to take on new challenges;
* Having good experiences at school—the prospect of this is increased with family engagement with the school and teachers and helping the child cope with schoolwork;
* Being accepted by peers—engagement in sporting activities and teams can lead to a sense of mutual achievement and optimism;
* Limiting exposure to risk—monitoring peer relationships and maintaining rules and boundaries. This is a particular area where parents may need encouragement. When exhausted and guilty it is easy to allow rules and standards to slip. Drug abuse, unsafe sex, and delinquency all can lead to negative chain reactions;
* Having some chores and roles at home—negotiated as far as possible and within the child's capacity—builds confidence and pride in having contributed.

Helping Parents Respond to the Hardest Question

If a child asks their parent if they are going to die, it is instinctive to offer reassurance, which in turn risks inhibiting the child from being able to express their fears. Parents benefit from having the tools to be able to respond in a way which doesn't crush the child's hope while maintaining their ability to talk openly. Examples of how a parent could respond include:

* *"Well, some people with cancer live for a very long time. I would like to be one of those people. But sometimes it doesn't work out and people might only live for a short time. That makes me sad. Is that something you want to talk about?"*

- *"I am doing everything I can do to be well, and the doctors are helping me as much as they can. I guess we can't always be sure how it might work out even though we are doing our best. What do you think about it all?"*
- *"I guess it is possible. That makes me so sad because I want to be with you. No matter what happens you are loved, and I will do my best to make sure you are safe."*

Need for Specialist Referral

Although tempting to consider that every bereaved child would benefit from specialist intervention, there is limited evidence to justify this approach. Bereavement is hard, but it is not an illness. Referral of a child can convey the message that the situation is so dreadful that it cannot be handled at home, or that the child has trouble coping. In addition, advocating for referral can be a means for some parents to avoid the challenging task of sharing their child's distress and having to confront their own grief. Referral should be considered if there is a marked change in the child's behavior from usual, either the development of new behaviors or exacerbation of usual behavior.

There are some instances in which a child and/or family may benefit from specialist referral. In the case of Janice above, her son Jock demonstrated behavior disturbance that was suggestive of a diagnosis of ADHD. Untreated, this would not only lead to distress for Jock but could compromise his longer-term outcome as he faced possible removal from his grandparents' care into an institution. In Jock's case it is highly likely that the distress about his mother's death compounded his behavior disturbance due to ADHD.

Table 8.1 Practical Strategies for Parents

Things That Will Likely Help	Things That Probably Won't
Talking	Keeping secrets
Maintaining routine	Letting go of structures and rules
Negotiating tasks	Giving orders
Telling children it is not their fault	Telling children to "be good for Mummy and Daddy"
Encouraging children to participate in sport and normal activities	Expecting children to spend all of their time at home "because time together is precious"
Giving information in stages	Talking about possible outcomes far into the future
Allowing others to offer support	Feeling that accepting help is weak or will lead to loss of independence
Letting children talk about difficult things	Rushing to reassure
Encouraging children to work out some problems themselves	Trying to fix everything for them
Letting the school know	Keeping everything private
Maintaining rules and consequences	Letting discipline slip because of guilt
Letting children see that parents are upset sometimes	Always adopting a façade and pretending everything is OK

The emergence of anxiety or depression also indicate the need for referral. Some children may be at increased risk because of a family history of mental illness. In these cases, parents should be encouraged to be aware of emerging symptoms. In young children, externalizing behaviors such as rough play and irritability may indicate anxiety or depression. Boys may be vulnerable because of socialization to be brave and avoid expression of emotions. The common admonition of a boy to "be the man of the house" after death of a father typically poses a burden and may result in distress manifest as marked behavior disturbance. This may attract criticism or even harsh discipline, which would in turn compound the child's distress. In adolescents, depression may be manifest as social withdrawal, feeling tired, and physical symptoms such as headaches and sleep disturbance. Expressions of guilt or low self-esteem always warrant further assessment.

There may be instances where referral does seem indicated, but the parent with support can identify and respond to their child's needs as illustrated in the following case history:

Case Study 2

Katrina was a 6-year-old girl whose father had metastatic colorectal cancer. Her mother was coping by focusing on practical issues and trying to not upset Katrina by talking about the situation. Over a period of several weeks Katrina had become more clinging and complained of feeling sick in the mornings. Her mother had kept her home from school on several occasions and had taken her to the family doctor who could not identify any medical condition to account for her symptoms. Katrina told her mother she did not want to go to her best friend's birthday party. She then refused to go on a school excursion. When her mother found her asleep on the floor outside the parent's bedroom, she was concerned that Katrina needed specialist help. With support from the clinic nurse the mother came to recognize that Katrina's behavior was designed to ensure proximity to her ill father. With gentle encouragement Katrina admitted she was afraid that "something bad would happen and she wouldn't know if she wasn't at home." The mother assured Katrina that if anything happened, no matter how small, she would immediately contact the school, or her friend's parents and bring her home, and there would be no secrets. Katrina's anxiety quickly abated.

Psychological Therapies/Practical Strategies for Children and Families

For children who have experienced parental death, there is emerging evidence that even brief interventions may reduce the risk of children developing depression. A range of formats are advocated however parental support and engagement are central with the aim of maximizing parental ability to support their children. A stepped care approach is advocated to supporting children living with parental cancer and following parental death, with the level of intervention based on family- and child-based vulnerability factors. Attention should be given to practical elements particular to the needs of young families such as finances and childcare support bearing in mind the vulnerability for single-parent families if there is financial strain or limited social support. When offering referral for specialist help, one always needs to be mindful of addressing any stigmatized attitudes and misconceptions vis-à-vis such help.

Interventions for All Families

Information

The most basic intervention is provision of information and support for parents and children. Health professionals are well placed to give information about children's responses and needs. However, parents who are under duress may not recall all information given verbally even over successive consultations, so it is valuable to supplement face-to-face information with a range of high-quality resources, many of which are available online free of charge. Having a tangible resource can be comforting for parents who can refer to the information repeatedly. Themes that are typically addressed include talking to children about cancer, children's reactions (age-specific), helping children and teenagers cope, explaining cancer treatments, and dealing with changes to family life. Although the focus for many is on early-stage disease there are resources focused on terminal disease as listed in the Additional Resources section at the end of the chapter. A range of children's books are good resources to talk about the topic of death and dying, particularly with younger children. Dolls, teddy bears, and drawings can help parents give explanations as well as give the child an opportunity to express their feelings. There are guides addressed to teens to help them understand and cope with cancer, changes in the family, and interactions with peers. Ideally these resources are accessed well before parental death to prepare children, and then provide ongoing benefit after bereavement.

Reminding the parent about how to recognize distress and encouraging children to talk about their concerns is important. Parents need to understand that adolescents may vary considerably in their expression of grief, vacillating between intense outward displays of distress, withdrawal, or seeming indifference to the situation. The grieving parent who fails to appreciate this can respond angrily to the adolescent, accusing them of not caring about the death and this in turn increases family tension and undermines coping.

Looking into the Future

It may be beneficial for parents to engage in a legacy project such as writing letters for future milestones of their children, compiling a photo album with narratives of special moments shared throughout their lives together, creating a book of family recipes as a generational hand-down to continue family traditions, or putting together a *legacy box* filled with objects of significance to the parent–child dyad and family. Parents can engage their children in discussions involving the sharing of meaningful events in their lives, life lessons learned, and advice moving forward. These need to be broached sensitively. It is important that a parent who does not want or feel able to do this is not made to feel that they are letting their child down. Similarly, maintaining a sense of connection with the deceased parent and incorporating remembrances into family life can be important ways to assist children, but the surviving parent who feels guilty or is overwhelmed will need support to maintain this connection for their children. It is important to include children in community rituals (e.g., funerals, unveiling of a gravestone or memorial plaque) while providing them with simple explanations as to their meaning, preparing them ahead of time, and being attentive to them during the event.

Maximizing Social Support
During the final stages of illness families may experience considerable practical and emotional support. In the months after death this support typically evaporates as friends and extended family resume their former life, often making assumptions that the bereaved family is "moving forward." A surviving parent may feel especially isolated during this time and struggle to mobilize supports, so this requires particular focus and practical suggestions. Conversely the surviving parent may feel that they should "just get on with it," but it is likely to be helpful for them to accept some practical assistance in daily life such as collecting children from school, help with homework, and taking children to sporting activities.

Engaging with the School
Involving the school is advocated to ensure they understand how the struggles at home may reflect in problematic behaviors at school, make readjustments to the academic schedule accordingly, foster nurturing connections to peers and teachers, and advise parents of any difficulties arising. Ideally, the parent would be coached to approach the school themselves and adolescents consulted in the decision with their wishes discussed and respected. Some schools may provide specialized support in the form of a school nurse, social worker, or psychologist. Oncology professionals supporting the parent and family can only approach the school with written parental consent, as well as consent of the adolescent once a certain age is reached. There are workbooks to support school staff in such circumstances, covering how the cancer diagnosis of a parent can affect a student and ways that the school can support the student and their family (see Additional Resources at the end of this chapter).

Interventions for Families with Greater Needs
For children and families with greater needs a more structured intervention may be considered. Consistent themes of well-evaluated interventions are facilitation by experienced health professionals such as psychologists or social workers who provide psychoeducation and supportive discussions for parents.

Box 8.3 Helpful Management Strategies

- Including significant family members and friends in ongoing "normal" activities can help children to feel more optimistic and confident.
- In addition, adults known to the child can be helpful in identifying any signs of distress in children.
- Adolescents, in particular, may be wary of expressing their grief for fear of overwhelming their parent.
- Having a supportive listener who is not the parent can be helpful.

Box 8.4 Core Topics in Psychoeducation

• Impact of a cancer diagnosis on the family and typical reactions of children
• Coping strategies
• Communication skills
• Maintaining a strong social network

Some parents come to the diagnosis of cancer with limited parenting skills due, for example, to their own childhood experiences of adversity, trauma, and mental health conditions. In a safe and supportive context parents can reflect on their own response to the cancer and be encouraged to consider their children's needs separately. Guidance and support can be provided to help parents to regulate their own emotional distress and learn strategies to be responsive to their children. Such programs are not widely available and rely on highly skilled professionals.

Considering the important role of family functioning affecting children's distress during parental cancer, one may also consider *formal family grief therapy*. Several models of such therapy exist, one is listed in Additional Resources. Family interventions can be particularly important to offer to at-risk families. Attention should be paid to anticipatory grief and the potential for a crisis moving forward, such as the presence for example of suicidal thoughts in the surviving parent or in adolescents.

Professional Issues and Service Implementation

There are few aspects of cancer care likely to engender more powerful emotions in patients and health professionals than responding to pending parental death when dependent children are involved. A range of complex issues may arise, and the following examples are presented to stimulate health professionals to reflect on the range of variables that can impact on outcome.

Recording and Communicating

Care in oncology is typically delivered in the context of a multidisciplinary team in which the expertise of a range of professionals contributes to optimal outcomes. Consent to treatment may be seen as tacit consent for sharing of information, however it is appropriate to explicitly discuss the nature of information that will be recorded and shared, respecting confidentiality about highly sensitive issues. Depending on the clinical service, there is a risk of fragmentation of care, for example if the parent is seen by a psychologist who works in another building or even different campus from the main oncology team. Electronic medical records ideally ensure that information is shared in "real time," however not all platforms are compatible. In many instances, written documentation of the outcomes of discussions and decisions (for example in a family meeting) needs to be supplemented with direct phone or face-to-face discussion to ensure that all team members are aligned with goals of care. This is critical if there are concerns about risk for children or parents.

Common Ethical Issues and Dilemmas

People facing life-limiting illness may make decisions that do not fit with what health professionals feel they would choose for themselves. Acknowledging and respecting the decisions of patients is essential, but this does not mean that there cannot be discussion about specific issues. For example, a parent may indicate that they do not want to discuss their illness with their child. Approaching this decision from a position of generosity and support rather than confrontation can lead to a shift in attitude. Initiating discussion with: "*I can see how much you love your children and would do anything to protect them. And I absolutely respect your decision.*" This could be followed with a suggestion framed as a question: "*I wonder if things don't go as well as we hope if there might be things that would be important to think about for the children? Maybe we can talk about this when we meet next.*" Ultimately the parent must decide on the way they wish to respond to their situation; however, health professionals should recognize that fear and helplessness are powerful drivers of avoidance and being nonjudgmental and offering hope are critical.

Cultural Issues

Treating those from different cultural backgrounds means recognition not just of language differences but also awareness of cultural understandings of illness and grief, and understanding of differing beliefs and rituals around death and dying (e.g., rituals to aid the soul's transition into the afterlife or to honor the dead, belief that the deceased can rise from the dead, grief behaviors such as loud outcries and slapping one's face, or dressing children in red at a funeral).

Opening discussion with a question such as "*What do I need to know about your culture and beliefs in order for me to give you the best possible care?*" can help. Language proficiency does not necessarily equate with health literacy, and health professionals should consider the use of plain English aids, one of which is noted in Additional Resources. Family members should not be used as interpreters and professional interpreters engaged. It can be useful to meet with the interpreter prior to a consultation to give some background, build rapport, and set goals. Professional interpreters can provide valuable insights into cultural beliefs about illness. (See Chapter 9 for more details on spiritual and culturally sensitive care).

Legal Issues

Recognition of the vulnerability of children with a parent who is dying from cancer is a core part of quality clinical care. A series of discussions with the family about their situation including practical issues and aspirations regarding care of children after parental death is required, ideally leading to mutual agreement. This may include appointment of a guardian and establishment of a trust to cover education and other costs. In some instances, tension and conflict regarding access to children can occur (for example a step-parent and biological parent who have different views). Negotiation of care arrangements requires input from skilled therapists such as social workers whose focus must be on the welfare of children. Unfortunately, in some instances there may be a need for legal involvement to protect children.

Teams and Supervision

Clinical supervision is a mechanism for health professionals to share details of their clinical experiences, patient management, and the emotional dimensions of their role in a safe and confidential environment. It aims to assist the health professional to gain greater insights into their professional roles and areas that may benefit from reflection or expanded learning. It is not a test or a way of finding fault or error. It is based on the premise that a more experienced practitioner can share information and support a less experienced practitioner to achieve the best outcomes for their patients and themselves. Supervision can be provided in a one-on-one setting or group setting. The role of the supervisor is to support and guide rather than giving instructions.

Clinical supervision is not a personal therapy and attendees do not generally discuss personal issues. However, there may be some occasions when this is relevant and useful. Faced with caring for a dying parent of dependent children there is the risk of over-involvement including self-disclosure and giving advice based on personal values. Boundary issues can arise, and patients may invite self-disclosure of their treating clinician. Many clinicians see some degree of self-disclosure as helpful in promoting rapport and trust. The clinician should always reflect on their motivation for disclosure (*Is it for them or is it for me?*) and recognize the potential for this to distort the professional relationship and even inhibit the patient from disclosing concerns. This could be to "protect" the clinician from their distress, or because they fear that they will be judged as not coping as well as the clinician who faced a similar situation.

A common question from parents who are facing death is to ask the clinician: "*Do you have children?*" This question is not necessarily a request for information about the clinician's family—it is more likely an expression of concern about whether the clinician grasps the enormity of their predicament. Declining to comment at all can be seen as churlish and disrespectful. A simple response such as "*Yes, I do. But I don't think anyone can really grasp the pain of the situation you are facing as a parent. What are the things that are worrying you the most as a parent?*"

References

1. Walczak A, McDonald F, Patterson P, Dobinson K. How does parental cancer affect adolescent and young adult offspring? A systematic review. Inter J Nurs Stud. 2017;77:54–80. https://doi.org/10.1016/j.ijnurstu.2017.08.017.

2. Morris J, Turnbull D, Preen D, Zajac I, Martini M. The psychological, social, and behavioral impact of a parent's cancer on adolescent and young adult offspring aged 10–24 at the time of diagnosis: A systematic review. J Adolescence. 2018;65:61–71. https://doi.org/10.1016/j.adolescence.2018.03.001.

3. Morris JN, Martini A, Preen D. The well-being of children impacted by a parent with cancer: An integrative review. Support Care Cancer. 2016;24(7):3235–3251. https://doi.org/10.1007/s00520-016-3214-2.

4. Lytje M, Dyregrov A. The price of loss—A literature review of the psychosocial and health consequences of childhood bereavement. Bereavement Care 2019;38(1):13–22. https://doi.org/10.1080/02682621.2019.1580854.

5. Ellis SJ, Wakefield C E, Antill G, Patterson P. Supporting children facing a parent's cancer diagnosis: A systematic review of children's psychosocial needs and existing interventions. Eur J Cancer Care. 2016; 26(1). https://doi.org/10.1111/ecc.12432. PMID: 26776913.

6. Alexander E, O'Connor M, Rees C, Halkett G. A systematic review of the current interventions available to support children living with parental cancer. Patient Educ Couns. 2019;102(10):1812–1821. https://doi:org/10.1016/j.pec.2019.05.001.

Further Reading

de Arruda-Colli MNF, Weaver M, Wiener L. Communication about dying, death, and bereavement: A systematic review of children's literature. J Palliat Med. 2017;20(5):548–559. https://doi.org/10.1089/jpm.2016.0494. This article gives details about story books written for children about the topics of dying and bereavement. Full titles and publication details are provided. Of note, the list includes books focusing on different ethnicities. It is likely to be a helpful reference for parents.

Kenyon BL. Current research in children's conceptions of death: A critical review. OMEGA—J Death Dying. 2001;43(1):63–91. https://journals.sagepub.com/doi/pdf/10.2190/0X2B-B1N9-A579-DVK1. Although an older article, this provides useful information for health professionals working with families about how children understand death.

Kissane DW, Bloch S. Family Focused Grief Therapy: A Model of Family-Centred Care during Palliative Care and Bereavement. Buckingham, UK: Open University Press; 2002. This text provides detailed information about the theoretical underpinnings of family therapy during palliative care and bereavement and is a useful resource for counselors.

Lewis FM, Brandt PA, Cochrane BB, et al. The Enhancing Connections Program: A six-state randomized clinical trial of a cancer parenting program. J Consult Clin Psych. 2015;83(1):12–23. https://doi.org/10.1037/a0038219. This publication describes the components of a parenting program for women with breast cancer, leading to benefits in parenting and depressed mood.

Additional Resources
Canadian Association of Psychosocial Oncology (CAPO). Start The Talk. https://startthetalk.ca/. Published 2018. Retrieved May 11, 2021. This resource consists of a series of modules about communicating with children and includes specific information for health professionals and educators.

Cancer Council. Cancer in the School Community—A Guide for Staff Members. https://www.cancervic.org.au/downloads/booklets/Cancer_in_the_School_Community/Cancer_In_The_School_Community.pdf. Published 2018. Accessed May 11, 2021. This resource includes practical information for teachers including how to respond when a staff member has cancer. There is information about preparation for death and planning a school memorial service.

Cancer Council. Talking to kids about cancer. A guide for people with cancer, their families and friends. https://www.cancer.org.au/assets/pdf/talking-to-kids-about-cancer-a-guide-for-people-with-cancer-their-families-and-friends Published 2018. Accessed January 11, 2021. This resource includes direct quotes from parents and children and has a section on communicating about advanced cancer.

Cancer Research UK. General Reading List—Supporting Children and Young Adults. https://www.cancerresearchuk.org/about-cancer/coping/general-books-links/general-reading-list. Published 2019. Retrieved May 11, 2021. This site provides links to a range of information about talking with children and more general issues related to cancer, treatment, and well-being.

Macmillan Cancer Support. Talking to Children When an Adult Has Cancer. https://www.youtube.com/watch?v=SrdQBZJ9bXk. Published 2012. Retrieved May 11, 2021. This video resource features Debbie, who talks about her children and the ways that she and her husband explained the diagnosis of breast cancer to the children. Her children ranged in age from teenage years to five years of age when she received the diagnosis.

Macmillan Cancer Support. Preparing a Child for Loss. https://books.google.ca/books?id=4ahxDwAAQBAJ&printsec=frontcover&source=gbs_ge_summar y_r&cad=0#v=onepage&q&f=false. Published 2021. Retrieved May 11, 2021. This resource focuses on bereavement and preparation of children for death of a loved one.

Macmillan Cancer Support. Talking to Children and Teenagers When an Adult Has Cancer. https://www.macmillan.org.uk/cancer-information-and-supp ort/stories-and-media/booklets/talking-to-children-and-teenagers-when-an-adult-has-cancer. Published 2019. Accessed January 11, 2021. This easy-to-read resource gives practical tips about talking with children and adolescents including their potential reactions and when to seek more specialized help.

National Cancer Institute. When Your Parent Has Cancer—A Guide for Teens. https://www.cancer.gov/publications/patient-education/when-your-parent-has-cancer Published 2012. Retrieved May 11, 2021. This resource is directed towards teenage children and includes narratives from teenagers and practical suggestions about coping and accessing support.

The Plain Language Thesaurus Version 3. National Centre for Disease Control and Prevention National Center for Health Marketing. https://www.orau.gov/ hsc/HealthCommWorks/MessageMappingGuide/resources/CDC%20Pl ain%20Language%20Thesaurus%20for%20Health%20Communication.pdf. Published 2007. Accessed January 14, 2021. This practical guide will be helpful for health professionals working across a range of clinical settings. It highlights the challenges that arise when a person has limited health literacy and provides suggestions to improve clarity of communication.

Chapter 9

Spiritually Sensitive Care in Palliative and End of Life Settings

Jayita Deodhar, Crystal Park, and Mark Lazenby

Learning Objectives

After reading this chapter, the clinician will be able to:

1. Describe the importance of spiritual care for patients receiving palliative or end of life care.
2. Understand the clinical presentations of patients carrying spiritual distress and be able to use a spiritual assessment tool to identify these spiritual concerns.
3. Describe key differential diagnoses and assessment approaches to ensure an optimal understanding of each patient's and family's spiritual and cultural needs.
4. Understand clinical, psychotherapeutic, or complementary interventions appropriate to patients' spiritual concerns and be able to refer for specialist care as appropriate.
5. Understand professional, legal, ethical, training, and service development issues that will enhance spiritually sensitive care.

Background

Spiritual concerns—worries or unease about spiritual matters—are commonly experienced in the context of cancer and can cause substantial distress and impair quality of life.[1] Thus, spiritual care is considered a standard component of cancer care in national and international palliative care guidelines.[2,3]

Spirituality is a broad and difficult-to-define concept; thus, "spiritual concerns" is an umbrella term encompassing many different existential as well as religious concerns. Spirituality can be defined variously as one's connection to the transcendent or the divine, as the connections between oneself and others, or even as the connection to one's deepest self. Spirituality also includes issues of meaning and purpose; it can be thought of as the way individuals answer existential questions. Although often expressed in

Box 9.1 Definition of Spirituality

Spirituality is a dynamic and intrinsic aspect of humanity through which individuals seek ultimate meaning, purpose, and transcendence, and experience relationship to self, family, others, community, society, nature, and the significant or sacred. Spirituality is expressed through beliefs, values, traditions, and practices.

Adapted from Ferrell BR, Twaddle ML, Melnick A, Meier DE. National Consensus Project Clinical Practice Guidelines for Quality Palliative Care Guidelines, 4th ed. J Palliat Med. 2018;21(12):1684–1689. https://doi.org/10.1089/jpm.2018.0431.

religious ways, spirituality is not always about religion. In the United States, the National Consensus Project for Quality Palliative Care has adopted a definition of spirituality in the context of palliative care as shown in Box 9.1.[3]

Cancer patients commonly report that religiousness and spirituality are important to them in dealing with their illness, relying on such resources as their personal relationship with God, or their religious community, to help them manage their distress. They often engage in religious or spiritual rituals such as prayer or meditation as efforts to cope. Religious and spiritual resources are typically associated with better adjustment to and coping with cancer as well as to better mental and physical health-related quality of life.[4] Thus, spiritual concerns may threaten patients' health and well-being and are an important focus of clinical care.

In the context of cancer, common spiritual concerns include fears about dying and about whether there is an afterlife, feeling angry with God for one's illness, questioning the power of God, or even feeling like the cancer is punishment for wrongs they may have committed. Other spiritual concerns are less about struggle and more about trying to deepen one's spirituality, such as seeking a closer connection with God or one's faith. Forgiveness is a common spiritual concern for cancer patients.[1] Some patients feel guilt and desire to be forgiven for wrongdoing, either by another individual or by God, while others feel a need to forgive a wrongdoing or repair an interpersonal schism.[5]

Cancer patients also often focus on meaning, both of the cancer and more broadly of their lives as a whole. Finding meaning in one's cancer experience may involve trying to determine why they became ill or finding some ways to use the illness in a positive way, such as devoting their suffering to God or being an example to others.[6] More broadly, it is common to contemplate the meaning of one's life; whether one has sufficiently had purpose, understood the world and one's place in it, and mattered to others or to the world at large.[7] Spiritual concerns can be religious, such as losing one's faith or desiring to deepen one's faith, and may be culturally specific to particular religions. For example, one study found that cancer patients who were Hindu expressed spiritual concerns regarding the benefits of Pooja, the concept of rebirth, and the belief in karma.[8]

Prevalence of Spiritual Concerns

Spiritual concerns are quite prevalent. In one study of advanced cancer patients, most patients (86%) endorsed at least one spiritual concern; the median number of spiritual concerns endorsed was four.[1] Younger patients expressed more spiritual concerns, and the number expressed was inversely associated with poorer psychological and physical quality of life.[1] Another study reported that while only 15% directly sought spiritual care, nearly 62% identified at least one spiritual concern.[9] Common concerns were unmet existential needs (fear of the dying process 32%; loss of control 31%), regret (20%), need for forgiveness (17%), guilt (13%), loss of hope (13%), and meaning (15%).[9] Eleven concerns were present for more than 10% of the participants and one-quarter of religiously orientated participants expressed >4 concerns.[9] The majority of palliative care patients feel that their health care providers should consider spiritual concerns within the medical setting. Spiritual concerns have also been noted as common in secular cultures.[10, 11]

Studies of cancer patients' spiritual concerns have focused primarily on advanced or end-stage disease, apparently assuming that spiritual concerns are primarily relevant at the end of life. On the contrary, spiritual concerns are experienced by patients with localized and less advanced cancers, cancer survivors, and caregivers.[12] In their meta-analysis, Ripamonti and colleagues[13] found that health-status variables (e.g., diagnosis, type and stage of disease, metastasis, time since current diagnosis, Karnofsky index) were not associated with levels of spiritual concerns, suggesting that spiritual concerns are common throughout the cancer continuum.

Culturally and Spiritually Sensitive Palliative Care

Understanding the human dimension of suffering entails exploring and managing patients' emotional, social, and spiritual concerns. Thus, delivering culturally and spiritually sensitive cancer care is an essential role of all palliative, hospice, and end of life services. While the cultural sensitivity is the responsibility of all team members, pastoral care and chaplaincy services may play a more dominant role in addressing religious concerns, while psycho-oncology providers bring greater experience in responding to psycho-existential issues and concerns. Delineating which team members are needed for certain patients and their families can be a noteworthy challenge.

Attention to cultural traditions alongside religious beliefs is essential to deliver person-centered care. These traditions might include the levels of family involvement when communicating about an illness and its management, understanding any key lay or folk beliefs about illness causation (e.g., beliefs about contagion that may limit social support in some cultures), cultural mores relating to preparation of the deceased body, sensitivity about any language barriers, communication with migrants and refugees, proper use

---

Box 9.2 Definition of Culturally Sensitive Care

In culturally sensitive care, a clinician responds appropriately to the customs, beliefs, feelings, or circumstances of a group of people that share a common and distinctive racial, ethic, linguistic, religious or cultural heritage.

Adapted from Department of Health US, Office of Minority Health (OMH). National Standards for Culturally and Linguistically Appropriate Services in Health Care: Executive Summary. Washington, DC: [March 2001]. http://minorityhealth.hhs.gov/assets/pdf/checked/executive.pdf.

of professional interpreters, and how clinicians need to respond to CALD—culturally and linguistically diverse—communities.

Understanding Suffering

Various models of care have conceptualized the domains of suffering experienced by patients and their caregivers. Suffering can arise from a threat to the wholeness of the person, where the many losses associated with illness reduce capacity and functioning, introducing the experience of frailty and human confrontation with the limits of life, its finite nature and the prospect of life ending. Palliative care usually adopts a symptom orientation to understand these changes in well-being. The doyen of psychosomatic medicine, George Engel, introduced the biopsychosocial model as a broader conceptual approach.

The primary elements of the biopsychosocial-spiritual model allow for understanding spirituality, including measuring and assessing it, and as such provide structure for delivering culturally and spiritually sensitive care.[14] According to Sulmasy,[15] spirituality is the person's relationship with a transcendent entity and can be practiced by connection to nature, social relationships, and individual beliefs, a definition close to the one adopted by the National Consensus Project on Quality Palliative Care.[3] Although it is different from religion, which is a set of beliefs of a group or community in search of connection with the transcendent, it can be expressed through religious practices, too.

The diagnosis of a serious illness disrupts a person's inner world and relationship with the external environment, affecting one's connection to transcendence. This disequilibrium brings about questions regarding meaning, purpose, relationships, and value. Illness is a "disruption" to the ordinary trajectory of life and, therefore, holistic care should aim at alleviating these disruptions. Hope, dignity and forgiveness are useful concepts in providing spiritual care. Palliative care professionals and cancer-care clinicians, hence, have a responsibility to understand a patient's spiritual history alongside their cultural background and address a patient's needs accordingly.

Cultural and Spiritual Differences

Although one of the goals of palliative care is to alleviate suffering, in some cultural and spiritual traditions, from Western monotheistic traditions to eastern karmic traditions, suffering can be considered redemptive. In these cases, psycho-oncology and palliative care professionals should seek to help patients and families identify what can be done to alleviate unwanted suffering, while accepting the spiritual significance of suffering in general. Some of the unwanted suffering may arise from feelings of shame or guilt, which can be covalent with the belief in redemptive suffering, especially in theological traditions in which such suffering expiates for past sins. In these cases, focusing on forgiveness can be a way forward.[15] As well, when patients feel shame or guilt, they may not wish to disclose their diagnosis of cancer very widely, including to some family members and to their communities of faith. In these instances, the psycho-oncology and palliative care teams can be a primary source of spiritual care.

Other cultural and spiritual differences include the unit of decision-making and care. In the West, with its emphasis on a personal deity in whose image one is created, the individual is, as with God, seen as the unit of decision-making, and thus, the unit of care. This idea of the autonomy of the self, while important for not violating a person's individual rights, can conflict with traditions in which the unit of decision-making is broader, including, for instance, one's family, one's elders, or one's children. The patient may turn to these broader networks for decision-making, as they may be spiritually invested with safeguarding the patient. In these cases, spiritual care becomes a communal, rather than an individual, affair. Many of the interventions that have been developed and tested come from cultural and spiritual traditions in which psycho-oncology and palliative care professionals are concerned about the individual patient. Some interventions have included caregivers,[16] but more interventions that focus on the broader context of spiritual support are needed.

The Efficacy of Spiritual and Existential Interventions

Evidence is building that spiritually and existentially oriented interventions enhance well-being. Engaging in religious practices generally improves adjustment to cancer, with a greater sense of meaning and purpose, improved self-care and support for family and carers.[17] Meaning-centered psychotherapy, dignity therapy, and life-review interventions enhance meaning and overall well-being.[18,19] There is still much work to do in demonstrating the benefits of spiritually directed care toward the end of life, but the evidence is mounting steadily.[20]

Presenting Problems

Patients with serious, life-limiting illness have spiritual needs and concerns, which if unaddressed, can impede care planning. Patients may present with emotional upheaval in the context of diagnosis of a serious illness, questioning God or doubting their meaning in life and purpose, and feeling lost and angry. The palliative care team and cancer-care clinicians collectively have the responsibility to explore these issues in the context of the patient's history, as the focus ought to be on holistic, person-centered, culturally competent care. Several authors have noted some barriers to this process, namely clinicians' discomfort in addressing spiritual issues, lack of training and structured protocols.

Some of the typical symptoms that patients may present with include:

- Dismay, existential angst, despair
- Religious doubts
- Loss of faith
- Guilt, regret
- Fear of punishment
- Prayers unheard
- Anger at God
- Need for forgiveness

- Conflict
- Struggle with uncertainty
- Sense of the pointlessness of life

Assessment

Assessment of spiritual needs is based on measurable domains. Four aspects have been described:

1. *Religiosity*: this covers aspects of spiritual beliefs, belonging to a particular religious community, and personal religious rituals practiced.
2. *Spiritual or religious coping*: this refers to how the individual's spiritual/religious beliefs and practice help in coping with a serious illness and imminent death.
3. *Spiritual well-being*: a quality of life marker, with the presence of spiritual distress negatively impacting the individual.
4. *Spiritual needs, issues, or concerns*: these are important to both assess and respond to, especially at the end of life.

Based on these domains, questions can be asked for screening, history-taking, and/or assessment. An inquiry based on these methods can direct interventions and referrals for specialist spiritual care.[21] This approach can be followed across different cultures and communities.

⚲ Screening

Key questions[18] include:

1. Whether religiosity or spirituality is important to the patient for coping with serious illness.
2. Whether religious or spiritual needs are being met by the care provided.
3. Whether the patient is at peace.[22] This single question can determine if the person is in crisis and, if so, prompt intervention becomes possible.

Also, the National Cancer Comprehensive Network's (NCCN) Distress Thermometer and Problem Check List has spiritual or religious concerns as a screening question, along with physical, emotional, family, social and practical concerns.[19]

Box 9.3 Importance of Spiritual Assessment

Cancer-care institutions in the United States that are accredited by the Joint Commission International are required to perform spiritual assessments of patients who are receiving end f life care. It is similar in other nations.

Adapted from The Joint Commission. Spiritual Beliefs and Preferences—Evaluating a Patient's Spiritual Needs. The Joint Commission Standards Website. https://www.jointcommission.org/standards/standard-faqs/hospital-and-hospital-clinics/rights-and-responsibilities-of-the-individual-ri/000001669 Accessed March 16, 2021.

⚲ Spiritual History Taking

Spiritual history-taking should be part of the comprehensive assessment of the patient, which helps the palliative care clinician or team member to understand the patients' experience of spirituality, any change in their spiritual belief systems in the context of their illness, their needs, and sources of spiritual/religious support.

↙ Key Assessment Tools

Several tools have been used for spiritual history taking, of which the FICA tool (see Box 9.4), developed by Puchalski,[23] and the HOPE tool (see Box 9.5), developed by Anandarajah and Hight,[24] are the two most commonly used.

There are other published approaches to spiritual assessment, including the SPIRIT assessment tool,[25] which includes components of an individual's spiritual belief, personal spirituality, presence of integration with community, rituals and practice, implications for organizing care, and planning for terminal events. These assessment tools have been developed and researched in the Western world with mainly White populations and may not translate well across all cultures. The FICA tool has been translated into three European languages. Also, most assessment tools have been used in research and hospice settings. Hence, clinicians need to be aware and appropriately phrase these questions in a culturally sensitive manner. Also, these prompts can help physicians, nurses, social workers, psychologists, and other members of palliative care teams to encourage patients to reflect on how their spiritual beliefs can improve their coping.

Box 9.4 FICA Spiritual Assessment Tool

F: *What is your faith or belief?*
• Do you consider yourself spiritual or religious?
• What things do you believe in that give meaning to your life?

I: *Is it important in your life?*
• What influence does it have on how you take care of yourself?
• How have your beliefs influenced your behavior during this illness?
• What role do your beliefs play in regaining your health?

C: *Are you part of a spiritual or religious community?*
• Is this of support to you and how?
• Is there a person or group of people you really love or who are really important to you?

A: *How would you like me, your healthcare provider, to address these issues? your healthcare?*

Adapted from Puchalski CM. The FICA Spiritual History Tool #274. J Palliat Med. 2014;17(1): 15–106. https://doi.org/10.1089/jpm.2013.9458

Box 9.5 HOPE Approach to Spiritual Assessment

H: Spiritual resources

• What are your sources of hope and peace?

O: Organized religion

• Are you a member of an organized religion?

• What religious practices are important to you?

P: Personal spirituality

• Do you have spiritual beliefs separate from organized religion?

• What spiritual practices are most helpful to you?

E: Effects on care

• Is there any conflict between your beliefs and the care you will be receiving?

• Do you hold beliefs or follow practices that you believe may affect your care?

• Do you wish to consult with a religious or spiritual leader when you are ill or making decisions about your healthcare?

Adapted from Anandarajah G, Hight E. Spirituality and medical practice: Using the HOPE questions as a practical tool for spiritual assessment. Am Fam Physician. 2001;63(1):81–89.

Referral for Specialist Spiritual Assessment

Spiritual assessment is a formal and detailed evaluation of the person's spiritual needs and resources that takes place in a narrative shared by the patient. This assessment is a specialized examination undertaken by trained spiritual care professionals. Components include meaning, grief and despair and the concept of forgiveness. A specialized model called the PC-7 has been developed by a group of chaplains involved in palliative care.[26] It is a quantifiable measure focusing on suffering, meaning, relationships, integrity, legacy, decision-making and spiritual-religious struggle or conflict.[23]

Subsequent to an assessment of patient's spiritual needs, the cancer-care clinicians and the palliative care team should incorporate these elements into the patient's overall care, thus better understanding and addressing the patient's suffering.

Diagnosis

A categorical structure for diagnosis of spiritual distress is not feasible. However, some guidelines have suggested concerns about the following states of life:

• Loss of meaning and purpose in life;

• The role of conflicts with one's own beliefs, community, or physicians;

• The loss of faith and hope;

• Guilt; and

• Grief.

Deep distress can develop from the inability to incorporate meaning and purpose in life, or the experience of loss of faith and connection to self, nature, or a higher power. Challenges can arise when people confront some of the very givens of human nature, such as death itself, our fundamental aloneness, our freedoms with the related responsibility, and the very meaning of life itself. *Of critical importance is the possibility that existential distress can increase the severity of depression and may lead to a desire for hastened death.*

Investigations for Key Differential Diagnoses

- *Major Depressive Disorder:* The diagnosis of Major Depressive Disorder (MDD), according to the 5th edition of *Diagnostic and Statistical Manual of Mental Disorders* (DSM-5), requires the patient to endorse at least five of nine symptoms for most of the day during the same two-week period: depressed mood; loss of interest or pleasure; weight loss or gain; disturbances in sleep; psychomotor agitation or retardation; fatigue; inability to concentrate; feelings of worthlessness or excessive guilt; and repeated suicidal thoughts (see also Chapter 4).

  At least one of the five symptoms must be either depressed mood or loss of interest or pleasure. Guilt, as experienced in spiritual distress, may be present but other diagnostic criteria that cause significant subjective distress or impact socio-occupational functioning must be endorsed by the patient for the diagnosis of MDD, which can be a single episode or recurrent. Consider use of the PHQ-9 as a measure of depression, whose score will be ≥ 10 when clinically significant.

- *Mood Disorders Secondary to Medical Conditions:* Consider comorbid states illustrated by endocrine disorders (e.g., hypothyroidism), neurological disorders (e.g., Parkinson's, stroke), autoimmune disorders (e.g., lupus), medication-induced disorders (e.g., steroids, opioids, anticancer therapies), malignant diseases (e.g., cytokines, paraneoplastic), and organ failures (e.g., liver, renal). Several investigations may need to be considered here through consultation with an appropriate physician.

- *Demoralization:* This incorporates loss of meaning and purpose, hopelessness, feeling trapped and discouraged, poor coping, and sense of failure, which can lead to suicidal thinking (see also Chapter 3). Consider use of the DS-II, whose score will be ≥8 when clinically significant. It can be present in patients with serious medical illnesses such as cancer, as well as in psychiatric disorders. Demoralization can lead to poor outcomes and desire for hastened death.

- *Anxiety disorders:* These are characterized by worry, fear and anxiety and are associated with behavioral manifestations (see also Chapter 2). Anxiety can be episodic (panic disorder), generalized (generalized anxiety disorder), or related to certain objects or situations (phobias). Consider use of the GAD-7, whose score will be ≥10 when clinically significant.

Clinical Management

A key clinical judgment is the selection of an appropriate intervention from what follows, tailored to the needs of the patient as a person.

Religious Interventions

Religious interventions include engaging in rites and practices, such as prayer, fasting, recitation of sacred texts, rituals of being anointed, having one's sins forgiven or taking communion, meditation, veneration of saints, departed loved ones, and the like.

🔍 *A key part of the clinical management of patients experiencing spiritual concerns is referral to professional spiritual care resources, such as chaplaincy.* However, not all institutions have professional spiritual care resources, and in some parts of the world, they are not standard of care. In these instances, making connections with the patient's spiritual community can be helpful, as spiritual or religious communities are often a source of spiritual care for cancer patients. Indeed, the third FICA assessment question is about whether the patient is a part of such a community.

However, not all spiritual people are part of spiritual or religious communities, and in many regions of the world, worship is not confined to a single place or community. For example, in some religions, such as Hinduism and Buddhism, worship can be performed in temples, at home, or even at shrines constructed in the workplace, and it may incorporate personal reflection, music, dance, or recitation of poetry. For these patients, being part of a singular spiritual or religious community may not be as helpful for spiritual support as their personal practices.

Psychotherapeutic Treatments

Meaning-Centered Psychotherapy

Meaning-centered psychotherapy (MCP) draws on a theoretical concept that each person has a drive to find and cultivate meaning in life, even as one's life may be coming to an end. Using a mix of didactics, in which the therapist introduces different concepts of meaning at the beginning of each session, and experiential exercises, in which patients explore sources of meaning in their lives, MCP is a psychoeducational approach.

The concepts the therapist explores include:

1. the meaning of life;
2. the desire to find meaning in human existence (the will to live); and
3. the freedom to find meaning in life, including when one suffers.

The sources of meaning the patient explores include:
- creative (engaging with life),
- experiential (connecting with life),
- attitudinal (turning life's limitations into triumphs), and
- historical (exploring legacy past, present, and future).

Table 9.1 describes the topics of MCP by weekly session. The individual format combines the third and fourth sessions into a single session, converting the model from eight group to seven individual sessions. For patients who are very near death, MCP has been adapted into a three-session intervention.[19,20]

Table 9.1 Meaning-Centered Psychotherapy by Weekly Session

Weekly Session	Session Topic	Session Content		
		Didactic	**Experiential Exercise**	**Homework**
1	Concepts and sources of meaning	Introductions; review of concepts and sources of meaning.	Meaningful moments	Read Frankl's *Man's Search for Meaning* and reflect on the question "Who am I?"
2	Cancer and meaning	Sense of identity before and after cancer diagnosis.	Who am I?	Reflect on the legacy one has been given (past).
3	Historical sources of meaning (past legacy), current sources of meaning (present) and future hopes (legacy)	Life as a legacy one has been given (past); life as a legacy one lives (present) and gives (future)	Historical sources of meaning (past); current sources of meaning and future hopes	Reflect on the legacy one lives (present) and gives (future); share one's story with someone and reflect on how one has encountered life's limitations
4	Attitudinal sources of meaning: encountering life's limitations	Confronting limitations imposed by cancer, prognosis, and death; introduction to legacy project	Encountering life's limitations	Reflect on creative sources of meaning
5	Creative sources of meaning: engaging in life fully	Creativity, courage, and responsibility	Creative sources of meaning	Reflect on experiences that have been sources of meaning
6	Experiential sources of meaning: connecting with life	Experiences as sources of meaning, such as love, nature, art, humor	Love, beauty, and humor	Complete a legacy project
7	Transitions: reflections and hopes for the future	Review sources of meaning as resources, reflect on lessons learned; and goodbyes	Hopes for the future	Share legacy project with family & friends

Adapted from Breitbart W, Pessin H, Rosenfeld B, et al. Individual meaning-centered psychotherapy for the treatment of psychological and existential distress: A randomized controlled trial in patients with advanced cancer: Individual Meaning-Centered Psychotherapy. Cancer. 2018;124(15):3231–3239. https://doi.org/10.1002/cncr.31539.

Acceptance and Commitment Therapy

A variant of cognitive-behavioral therapy, acceptance and commitment therapy's (ACT) goal is to change the function of problematic or distressing thoughts, rather than to change or adapt them. Acceptance, in ACT, is the active choice against avoiding thoughts, feelings, and emotions so as to be fully present with them in the moment. It is a willingness to have unwanted experiences, if these experiences are part and parcel of doing the things that matter to the individual.[27] In the context of cancer, ACT is concerned with patients' attempts at avoiding thoughts and experiences of suffering that cause patients to withdraw from that which matters to them.

The evidence base for ACT in cancer patients is still emerging, yet acceptance of an inescapable reality may prove helpful. For ACT, suffering arises in how patients are open to their experiences. Because suffering is a product of inner experience, it can be ameliorated by experiencing one's private world with openness and greater acceptance. ACT can help patients to access spiritual resources and create life meaning as well as aid in the resolution or transformation of spiritual struggles.

Dignity Therapy

Dignity therapy is based on the concept of generativity, namely, that individuals have the ability to reflect on life with a sense of having made a difference and invested psychological energy into the lives of those who will outlive them. It can involve brief (30- to 60-minute) sessions, in which the therapist or biographer asks a series of open-ended questions that encourage patients near the end of life to talk about their lives or what matters most to them (see Table 9.2). The conversation is recorded, transcribed, and edited. It is then returned to the patient within a few days. The patient reads the transcript and make changes before a final version is produced. The patient may share this final version with family and friends. In a randomized controlled trial, dignity therapy has been shown to improve patients' levels of dignity, and when compared with usual palliative care, it has been shown to decrease demoralization and desire for hastened death.[21]

Life Review or Biography

Life review, which aims to integrate positive and negative life events into a coherent life story, can be undertaken in 2–6 sessions in which patients are asked to reflect on eight questions (see Table 9.3). The life review intervention improved patients' spiritual well-being and psychological distress. A meta-analysis found that life review is potentially beneficial in alleviating psycho-spiritual distress in end of life cancer patients.[22] A recent trial of a life review intervention in cancer patients found evidence of improved spiritual well-being.[28] Many palliative care services have adopted this model as a biography service,[29] usually provided by trained volunteers, who record the life review sessions, type them up, and include photographs and other commemorative images into a document that honors the person's life. The biography is presented to the patient and the family and often quoted in eulogies at funerals.

Table 9.2 Dignity Therapy Protocol

Questions

- Tell me a little about your life history; particularly the parts that you either remember most or think are the most important?
- When did you feel most alive?
- Are there specific things that you would want your family to know about you, and are there particular things you would want them to remember?
- What are the most important roles you have played in life (family roles, vocational roles, community-service roles, etc.)?
- Why were they so important to you, and what do you think you accomplished in those roles?
- What are your most important accomplishments, and what do you feel most proud of?
- Are there particular things that you feel still need to be said to your loved ones or things that you would want to take the time to say once again?
- What are your hopes and dreams for your loved ones?
- What have you learned about life that you would want to pass along to others?
- What advice or words of guidance would you wish to pass along to your (son, daughter, husband, wife, parents, other[s])?
- Are there words or perhaps even instructions that you would like to offer your family to help prepare them for the future?
- In creating this permanent record, are there other things that you would like included?

Adapted with permission from Chochinov HM, Hack T, Hassard T, Kristjanson LJ, McClement S, Harlos M. Dignity therapy: A novel psychotherapeutic intervention for patients near the end of life. J Clin Oncol. 2005;23(24):5520–5525. https://doi.org/23/24/5520.

Table 9.3 Life Review Questions for Biography Volunteers

Questions

- What is the most important thing in your life and why?
- What are the most vivid or impressive memories in your life?
- In your life, what event or person affected you most?
- What is the most important role you played in your life?
- What is the proudest moment in your life?
- Is there anything about you that your family needs to know?
- Are there things you want to tell them and are there things you want them to remember?
- What advice or words of guidance do you have for the important people in your life or for the younger generation?

Adapted with permission from Ando M, Morita T, Akechi, T, Okamoto T. Efficacy of short-term life-review interviews on the spiritual well-being of terminally ill cancer patients. J Pain Symptom Manage. 2010;39(6):993–1002. https://doi.org/10.1016/j.jpainsymman.2009.11.320.

Psychedelic-Assisted Psychotherapy

Recent trials in patients with life-limiting cancer using psilocybin as a psychedelic to create an experience from which meaning can be derived psychotherapeutically have demonstrated reduced symptoms of demoralization, anxiety, depression, and existential distress. Another recent trial of 3,4-methylenedioxy-methylamphetamine (MDMA) suggests similar reductions in existential distress associated with life-limiting illness. While these agents may be promising in treating some of the spiritual dimensions of cancer-related distress, they are not yet approved for use in most countries around the world and thus remain experimental.

Complementary Therapies

Integrative medicine, sometimes referred to as complementary medicine, provides diverse approaches to alleviate discomfort and promote well-being that may be particularly useful in addressing spiritual concerns in the palliative care context. These approaches include mind-body practices such as meditation and yoga, energy healing (e.g., reiki), shamanism, and therapeutic art and music. Integrative medicine approaches can provide nonverbal, noncognitive methods for achieving peace and relaxation. Through experiencing these enhanced states, patients may gain greater insights and self-understanding, helping them to address their spiritual concerns.

Although integrative approaches are often included in palliative care, their use to specifically facilitate addressing spiritual concerns is not well documented.

- Mind-body practices appear particularly well suited to address spiritual needs, especially yoga.
- Yoga's potential for addressing spiritual concerns for patients in palliative care draws from its religious origins in ancient times and its direct applications to suffering. Yoga encompasses a strong philosophy of living (encompassing principles such as nonattachment and equanimity) as well as a set of powerful and easily taught practices that can have profound effects on calming both the central nervous system (e.g., breath regulation) and the mind (mindful awareness, gentle postures).

Care Available in the Community

Much of the literature available in spiritual assessment and interventions is restricted to research settings. Clinical work in this area is focused primarily on hospice care. Cultural differences between developed and developing nations are responsible for the lack of generalizability of spiritual assessment tools and interventions for spiritual care. Culturally appropriate tools for spiritual assessment in low- and middle-income countries have been developed; however, these studies have been conducted in tertiary care settings.[30] There is a paucity of studies on the spiritual care of cancer patients in community settings.

Professional Issues and Service Implementation

It is common in the West to have professional spiritual care providers on staff at hospitals or cancer centers. This mirrors the professionalization of the clergy or the availability of pastoral care training programs in these regions. However, not all cultural and spiritual traditions have such professional care providers. In some traditions, people are born into priestly roles, in which they function only at places of worship. In these traditions, the idea of receiving spiritual care at a hospital or cancer center may be at the very least odd, if not off-putting. *This notwithstanding, psycho-oncology staff can deliver spiritually and sensitive palliative care by using an appropriate assessment and intervention.*

Training in Spiritual Care

For delivery of compassionate person-centered care, clinicians need to be trained in identification, diagnostic assessment, and interventions, before delivering care. However, this professional balance can be difficult to navigate. Professionals have to be cognizant of their self-reflections and be aware of transference and countertransference issues. Oncology, psycho-oncology, and palliative care services and teams should develop and implement protocols for assessment and documentation while maintaining confidentiality. Triggers for referral to specialist services like pastoral care or chaplaincy should be established and implemented. Culturally appropriate spiritual care services need to be routine.

A significant barrier to providing culturally and spiritually sensitive palliative and end of life care is providers' discomfort with spirituality. Providers first must seek to heal themselves spiritually before they can offer spiritual care to others. One such way is through training.

An interprofessional curriculum on spiritual care has been developed by and implemented through the George Washington University Institute for Spirituality and Health (see Further Reading). This multidisciplinary curriculum includes modules on (1) spiritual distress, (2) compassionate presence, (3) spiritual assessments, (4) ethics and professional issues, and (5) the spirituality of healthcare professionals themselves. Other countries provide tertiary courses on pastoral care. Such education is critically important, as is the principle that healthcare professionals be self-aware and comfortable with their own spirituality.

Communication and Professional Relationships

A patient's and family's approach to palliative care, particularly to the end of life, should be honored and supported. Providers' need to form a compassionate, nonjudgmental, respectful relationship with patients and families, especially with regard to their cultural and spiritual approaches to cancer care. Respect means valuing patients' and families' views, even when they differ from more frequently encountered belief systems. Respect also extends to the recognition that, even if the provider and the patient and family are from the same religious tradition, they may not necessarily follow all practices and beliefs of that religion. Attempts at theological argument or conversion violate this respect.

Legal and Ethical Issues

Medical Aid in Dying

In some countries, euthanasia and clinician aid in dying, also called physician-assisted suicide, is legal, with qualifications. This can conflict with some providers' beliefs. While it can be seen as a morally complicated topic, psycho-oncology providers might first try one of the psychotherapies that has shown efficacy in addressing demoralization and desire for hastened death, such as dignity- or meaning-centered psychotherapy. Support for healthcare providers who develop moral distress will be a future need.

Other Ethical Challenges

Providers will meet a range of other issues, such as competing interests among members of a family, different attitudes toward the goals of care, different strengths of religious conviction, and adoption of advance care plans where values differ. Consultation with a clinical ethics service will sometimes be needed. Psycho-oncologists adopt a neutral stance as they support families in such predicaments.

Policies and Protocols

Most institutions will have formal policies around referral to pastoral care and chaplaincy services. These programs will usually be organized following a nondenominational spiritual model but will hold a register of accredited religious providers from multiple denominations to meet the needs of the local community, always cognizant of the needs of migrants and refugees as they join local communities.

References

1. Winkelman WD, Lauderdale K, Balboni MJ, et al. The relationship of spiritual concerns to the quality of life of advanced cancer patients: Preliminary findings. J Palliat Med. 2011;14(9):122–1028. https://doi.org/10.1089/jpm.2010.0536.

2. Connor SR, Gwyther E. The Worldwide Hospice Palliative Care Alliance. J Pain Symptom Manage. 2018;55(2S):S112–S116. https://doi.org/S0885-3924 (17)30360-3[pii].

3. Ferrell BR, Twaddle ML, Melnick A, Meier DE. National Consensus Project Clinical Practice Guidelines for Quality Palliative Care Guidelines, 4th Edition. J Palliat Med. 2018;21(12):1684–1689. https://doi.org/10.1089/jpm.2018.0431.

4. Thuné-Boyle IC, Stygall JA, Keshtgar MR, Newman SP. Do religious/spiritual coping strategies affect illness adjustment in patients with cancer? A systematic review of the literature. Soc Sci Med. 2006;63(1):151–164. https://doi.org/10.1016/j.socscimed.2005.11.055.

5. Riklikienė O, Spirgienė L, Kaselienė S, Luneckaitė Ž, Tomkevičiūtė J, Büssing A. Translation, cultural, and clinical validation of the Lithuanian version of the Spiritual Needs Questionnaire among hospitalized cancer patients. Medicina (Kaunas, Lithuania). 2019;55(11):738. https://doi.org/10.3390/medicina55110738.

6. Hall ME, Shannonhouse L, Aten J, McMartin J, Silverman E. Theodicy or not? Spiritual struggles of evangelical cancer survivors. J Psychol and Theol. 2019;47(4):259–277. https://doi.org/10.1177/0091647118807187.

7. Mesquita AC, Chaves, ÉCL, Barros, GAM. Spiritual needs of patients with cancer in palliative care: An integrative review. Curr Opin Support Palliat Care. 2017;11(4):334–340. https://doi.org/10.1097/SPC.0000000000000308.

8. Simha S, Noble S, Chaturvedi S. Spiritual concerns in Hindu cancer patients undergoing palliative care: A qualitative study. Indian J Pall Care. 2013;19(2):99–105. https://doi.org/10.4103/0973-1075.116716.

9. Michael NG, Bobevski I, Georgousopoulou E, et al. Unmet spiritual needs in palliative care: Psychometrics of a screening checklist. BMJ Support Palliat. 2020:1–7. https://doi.org/10.1136/bmjspcare-2020-002636.

10. Cheng Q, Xu X, Liu X, Mao T, Chen Y. Spiritual needs and their associated factors among cancer patients in China: A cross-sectional study. Support Care Cancer. 2018;26(10):3405–3412. https://doi.org/10.1007/s00 520-018-4119-z.

11. Hvidt NC, Mikkelsen TB, Zwisler AD, Tofte JB, Assing Hvidt E. Spiritual, religious, and existential concerns of cancer survivors in a secular country with focus on age, gender, and emotional challenges. Support Care Cancer.. 2019;27(12):4713–4721. https://doi.org/10.1007/s00520-019-04775-4.

12. Rabow MW, Knish SJ. Spiritual well-being among outpatients with cancer receiving concurrent oncologic and palliative care. Support Care Cancer. 2015;23(4):919–923. https://doi.org/10.1007/s00520-014-2428-4

13. Ripamonti CI, Giuntoli F, Gonella S, Miccinesi G. Spiritual care in cancer patients: A need or an option? Curr Opin Oncol. 2018;30(4):212–218. https://doi.org/10.1097/CCO.0000000000000454.

14. Sulmasy DP. A biopsychosocial-spiritual model for the care of patients at the end of life. Gerontologist. 2002;42 Spec No 3:24–33. https://doi.org/10.1093/geront/42.suppl_3.24.

15. Best M, Aldridge L, Butow P, Olver I, Price MA, Webster F. Treatment of holistic suffering in cancer: A systematic literature review. Palliat Med. 2015;29(10):885–898. https://doi.org/10.1177/0269216315581538.

16. Applebaum AJ, Buda KL, Schofield E, et al. Exploring the cancer caregiver's journey through web-based meaning-centered psychotherapy. Psycho-Oncology. 2018;27(3):847–856. https://doi.org/10.1002/pon.4583.

17. Goudarzian AH, Boyle C, Beik S, et al. Self-care in Iranian cancer patients: The role of religious coping. J Relig Health. 2019;58(1):259–270. https://doi.org/10.1007/s10943-018-0647-6.

18. Rosenfeld B, Saracino R, Tobias K, et al. Adapting meaning-centered psychotherapy for the palliative care setting: Results of a pilot study. Palliat Med. 2017;31(2):140–146. https://doi.org/10.1177/0269216316651570.

19. Wang C, Chow AYM, Chan CLW. The effects of life review interventions on spiritual well-being, psychological distress, and quality of life in patients with terminal or advanced cancer: A systematic review and meta-analysis of randomized controlled trials. Palliat Med. 2017;31(10):883–894. https://doi.org/10.1177/0269216317705101.

20. Puchalski CM, Sbrana A, Ferrell B, et al. Interprofessional spiritual care in oncology: A literature review. ESMO Open. 2019;4(1):e000465–000465. eCollection 2019.https://do.org/:10.1136/esmoopen-2018-000465.

21. Fitchett G. Assessing Spiritual Needs in a Clinical Setting. Website. http://www.ecrsh.eu/mm/Fitchett_-_Keynote_ECRSH14.pdf. Accessed March 16, 2021.

22. National Comprehensive Cancer Network. NCCN Clinical Practice Guidelines in Oncology Distress Management, Version 2.2021. NCCN Clinical Practice Guidelines in Oncology Website. https://www.nccn.org/profession als/physician_gls/pdf/distress.pdf. Accessed March 16, 2021.

23. Puchalski CM. The FICA spiritual history tool #274. J Palliat Med. 2014;17(1):15–106. https://doi.org/10.1089/jpm.2013.9458.

24. Anandarajah G, Hight E. Spirituality and medical practice: Using the HOPE questions as a practical tool for spiritual assessment. Am Fam Physician. 2001;63(1):81–89.

25. Ambuel B. Taking a spiritual history #19. J Palliat Med. 2003;6(6):932–933. https://doi.org/10.1089/109662103322654839.

26. Fitchett G, Hisey Pierson AL, Hoffmeyer C, et al. Development of the PC-7, a quantifiable assessment of spiritual concerns of patients receiving palliative care near the end of life. J Palliat Med. 2020;23(2):248–253. https://doi.org/10.1089/jpm.2019.0188.

27. Santiago PN, Gall TL. Acceptance and commitment therapy as a spiritually integrated psychotherapy. Counseling Values. 2016;61(2):239–254. https://doi.org/10.1002/cvj.12040.

28. Post L, Ganzevoort RR, Verdonck-De Leeuw IM. Transcending the suffering in cancer: Impact of a spiritual life review intervention on spiritual re-evaluation, spiritual growth and psycho-spiritual wellbeing. Religions (Basel, Switzerland). 2020;11(3):142. https://doi.org/10.3390/rel11030142.

29. Beasley E, Brooker J, Warren N, et al. The lived experience of volunteering in a palliative care biography service. Palliat Support Care. 2015;13(5):1417–1425. https://doi.org/10.1017/S1478951515000152.

30. Bhatnagar S, Noble S, Chaturvedi SK, Gielen J. Development and psychometric assessment of a spirituality questionnaire for Indian palliative care patients. Ind J Palliat Care. 2016;22(1):9–18. https://doi.org/10.4103/0973-1075.173939.

Further Reading

Ando M, Morita T, Akechi, T, Okamoto T. Efficacy of short-term life-review interviews on the spiritual well-being of terminally ill cancer patients. J Pain Symptom Manage. 2010;39(6):993–1002. https://doi.org/10.1016/j.jpai nsymman.2009.11.320. Classic paper on life-review interviews

Chochinov HM, Hack T, Hassard T, Kristjanson LJ, McClement S, Harlos M. Dignity therapy: A novel psychotherapeutic intervention for patients near the end of life. J Clin Oncol. 2005;23(24):5520–5525. https://doi.org/23/24/5520. Classic paper outlining dignity therapy as an intervention.

Lazenby M, McCorkle R, Sulmasy DP. Safe Passage: A Global Spiritual Sourcebook for Care at the End of Life. New York: Oxford University Press; 2014. This book coaches clinicians and others on the front lines of palliative and end of life care on understanding how to incorporate different cultural and spiritual traditions into the most difficult of moments around the end of life.

Paloutzian RF, Park CL. Handbook of the Psychology of Religion and Spirituality. 2nd ed. New York: Guilford Press; 2013. One of the author's textbook examining psychological dimensions of spirituality.

Puchalski C, Jafari N, Buller H, Haythorn T, Jacobs C, Ferrell B. Interprofessional spiritual care education curriculum: A milestone toward the provision of spiritual care. J Palliat Med. 2020;23(6):777–784. https://doi.org/10.1089/jpm.2019.0375. Recommended curriculum to train spiritual care providers.

Steinhorn DM, Din J, Johnson A. Healing, spirituality and integrative medicine. Ann Palliat Med. 2017;6(3):237–247. Overview of the interface between spirituality and integrative medicine in the setting of palliative care.

Chapter 10

Bereavement Care

Wendy G. Lichtenthal, William E. Rosa,
and Robert A. Neimeyer

Learning Objectives

After reading this chapter, clinicians will be able to:

1. Assess common grief reactions and risk factors for poor bereavement outcomes.
2. Adopt a family-centered approach to supporting grief and loss, thus ensuring continuity of care from cancer diagnosis, throughout illness, and into the bereavement phase.
3. Identify evidence-based grief interventions to normalize grief, educate families, and support adaptive coping responses.
4. Understand relevant professional, ethical, and cultural issues in supporting the bereaved after caring for palliative care patients.

Background Evidence

Bereavement care is a foundational aspect of quality palliative care in oncology settings. Access to high-quality palliative care is considered a human right by major organizations worldwide. Key components include providing support to the family and caregivers during the patient's illness and into bereavement, recognizing and respecting cultural values and beliefs of the patient and family, and supporting patients to live as fully as possible until death by facilitating effective communication that aids them and their families in determining goals of care. Without evidence-based and person-centered interventions that attend to grief and bereavement, palliative care services will consistently miss the mark.

Starting at the time of diagnosis and throughout the cancer trajectory, both patients and their families of choice will likely grieve a number of difficult losses, including changes to physical capacity and appearance, role identities, and future hopes and plans. Following the patient's death, grieving family members may not only intensely yearn for the patient, but they may also experience guilt, regret, and anger as they reflect on the patient's illness and end of life experiences. A significant subset of grieving family members may present with mental health challenges. Approximately 6 months following bereavement, studies of bereaved caregivers have shown the prevalence of:

- Major Depressive Disorder (MDD) ~6%;[1]
- Generalized Anxiety Disorder (GAD) ~2%[1]
- Panic Disorder (PD) ~3%;[1]
- Posttraumatic Stress Disorder (PTSD) ~3%;[1] and
- Prolonged Grief Disorder (PGD) ~8%.[2]

Psycho-oncology clinicians play a critical role in developing empathic, trusting relationships throughout the illness course to ensure care continuity from before to after the patient's death and to facilitate adaptive coping using a family-centered approach to palliative care. While the patient is alive, they can practice as "bereavement-conscious" clinicians; that is, they can engage in patient care with a mindfulness about the family's potential reactions after the patient's death, supporting emotional processing and helping to mitigate confusion, regrets, and guilt.[3] Clinicians may offer surviving family members both comfort and predictability by helping them to understand the dying process and providing psychosocial and emotional support following the patient's death.

Broadly speaking, psycho-oncology clinicians should be able to recognize the various presentations of grief, be familiar with risk factors for poor bereavement outcomes, and feel equipped to manage grief or make referrals for specialized grief interventions when warranted. On average, grief interventions appear to have small to moderate effects,[4] which is comparable to the effects of other psychotherapeutic interventions. One-on-one treatments targeting high-risk or symptomatic individuals, particularly those who are at least six-months post-loss, seem to yield stronger effects.[4]

This chapter will describe the clinical presentation of grief and related psychological reactions before and after a significant interpersonal loss, including considerations for making a differential diagnosis between typical grief and more concerning responses. It will also review interventions that can be applied to support the bereaved in the palliative care context.

There are several terms related to grief and bereavement used in the literature and by clinicians; these are detailed in Box 10.1 for reference. It is also helpful for psycho-oncologists to have familiarity with a range of bereavement theories, which can assist them with conceptualizing grieving family members' reactions and can provide a conceptual premise for helpful psychoeducation that can be woven into support efforts. The theories as well as intervention approaches that apply these theories are described in Table 10.1. They suggest adaptive tasks as well as potential strategies to prevent poor bereavement outcomes and reduce grief intensity.

Presenting Problems

Psycho-oncology clinicians providing palliative care will likely witness grieving in varied circumstances and contexts, including illness-related and anticipatory grief as disease progresses, acute grief surrounding the time of death,

---

Box 10.1 Definitions Related to Grief and Bereavement

- **Bereavement**: the *state of having experienced* a loss resulting from death
- **Grief**: the distressing *response* to any loss, including related feelings, cognitions, and behaviors
- **Mourning**: the *process of adapting to a loss*, which includes expression of grief and culturally, religious, and socially influenced behaviors, such as grieving rituals
- **Pre-death grief:** the distress and related emotions, cognitions, and behaviors *occurring before the patient's death*, including pre-loss grief and anticipatory grief
- **Anticipatory grief:** the separation distress and related emotions, cognitions, and behaviors *related to the patient's anticipated death*
- **Illness-related grief:** the distress and related emotions, cognitions, and behaviors related to losses occurring for the patient and family *in the here-and-now before the patient's death*, such as loss of physical functioning
- **Prolonged grief disorder:** a *distressing, disabling, and protracted grief reaction* characterized by intense and persistent yearning in addition to other severe symptoms, including avoidance, anger, identity challenges, and a sense of meaningless following a significant loss
- **Disenfranchised grief:** occurs with losses that are not recognized by society, resulting in *less social permission to express one's grief*

---

and in some cases, prolonged grieving that does not appear to improve over time. This section provides a summary of the presenting problems and important considerations associated with grief throughout the illness trajectory, including pathological responses to grief and specific, unique loss circumstances.

Pre-Death Grief

Those bereaved by cancer commonly begin grieving long before the death of their loved one. Starting at diagnosis, grief may emerge as the possibility of the patient's death is considered. If a poor prognosis is communicated to the patient and family, cognitive and emotional acceptance of the possibility of death is likely to be a nonlinear process; patients and families may both acknowledge the implications of the prognostic reality, while maintaining hope for a cure. Grief emerges in parallel, variably manifesting as:

- Sadness
- Anger
- Overt protest
- Increased protectiveness of the patient
- Separation anxiety

As feelings wax and wane, it is important to consider that both grief and hope can coexist.

Table 10.1 Theoretical Models of Grief

Theory	Key Concepts
Attachment Theory	• Attachment is instinctual for safety and security to promote survival. • Working models of early attachments, such as those between child and caregiver, are internalized. • Individuals with insecure attachment styles are at greater risk for separation distress and prolonged grief symptoms.
Evolutionary Theories	• Grief reactions encourage reunion when separated from attachment figures. • Grief signals to others that reorganization of relationships and goals is needed.
Psychodynamic Theories	• Early experiences influence reactions to loss and separation. • Yearning for the lost object is considered an adaptive response. • Adaptive processing of emotions occurs through "grief work".
Interpersonal Theories	• Patterns of interpersonal interactions and roles shape identity and self-schemas. • Adaptation involves integration of the relationship with the deceased and establishment of new (or deepening of existing) relationships.
Meaning Reconstruction Theories	• Adaptive grieving entails reaffirming or reconstructing mourners' narratives and meaning systems, which may be challenged by the loss when core assumptions are violated. • Adjustment to loss involves processing the event story of the death, realigning the back story of the relationship to the deceased, and revising the personal story of the mourner's identity in light of the loss.
Cognitive-Behavioral Theory	• Emotions, thoughts, and behaviors influence one another. • Maladaptive thoughts about the loss or deceased can result in anger, regret, guilt, and prolonged grief. • Avoidance of reminders of the loss and related emotions is negatively reinforcing and can interfere with processing of grief and with reengagement in adaptive experiences. • Third wave cognitive-behavioral theories consider how bereaved individuals think about and avoid vs. accept difficult emotional states.
Sociological Theories	• Society influences mourning, including cultural rituals and behaviors related to continued bonds with the deceased. • Culture and social norms affect individuals' sense of permission to express grief and acknowledge the loss. • Social support can reduce isolation, provide opportunities for grief processing, and buffer additional stressors in bereavement.

Table 10.1 Continued

Theory	Key Concepts
Family Systems Theory	• Bereaved family members impact one another's grief reactions. • Grief is impacted by the deceased's family role in the family. • The family's pre-loss level of functioning influences coping and adjustment to the loss.
Dual Process Model of Coping	• The process of adapting to loss involves oscillation between loss-oriented processes, which focus on confronting the pain and reality of the loss, and restoration-oriented processes, which focus on acclimating in the world without the deceased physically present and which provide respite from grief.
Task Model	• There are four core tasks involved in adapting to loss, including accepting the reality of the loss, working through the emotional pain of grief, adjusting to a world without the deceased physically present, and transforming the connection to the deceased.
Neurobiopsychosocial Theories	• Separation results in an acute stress response. • Grief involves activation of brain regions involved in emotion-focused memories (e.g., the posterior cingulate cortex) and reward centers (e.g., the nucleus accumbens).

There have been many terms to characterize *pre-death grief*, that is, grief occurring before the patient's death.[5]

- *Illness-related grief* may be used to characterize grief over losses in the "here-and-now," for example, as the patient loses their ability to function or fulfill role responsibilities. Such grief overlaps with but is distinct from anticipatory grief.
- *Anticipatory grief*, which manifests in response to contemplation of the patient's future death, reflects separation distress and is characterized by sadness and anxiety.[5] Heightened severity of anticipatory grief may be observed when evidence of disease progression is communicated to the patient and family. As the patient's death approaches, family members naturally will present with a range of intense emotions, including heightened grief and sadness as well as acute anxiety. They often focus exceptional attention on the patient's needs and well-being. Given how intensely their grief and anxiety may emerge, family members may at times have difficulty processing details of medical information communicated to them.[6] Predictors of more intense anticipatory grief include[7]*:
  - Inability to make sense of the pending loss
  - Relational dependency on the dying patient
  - Spiritual struggles

Higher levels of pre-death grief symptoms have been associated with both prolonged grief and depressive symptoms in bereavement.[5]

Acute Grief following the Death

The clinical presentation of acute grief in the weeks and months after the patient's death is highly individualized. Even within a given family system, the course and expression of acute grief varies; in fact, family members commonly regulate their feelings in response to how they perceive other members are coping. For example, one family member may not feel permission to express their grief because they do not want to further upset other members of the family. Another may feel the family is not expressing grief "enough" and may therefore feel compelled to be very open about their pain. Family members "coregulate" their emotion by silencing the expression of their personal grief to "protect" other family members, to safeguard their own private bond with the deceased, and to keep a manageable distance from the core pain of the loss.[8]

⚲ Key Message

The intense distress and associated emotions during the first months of bereavement following a death may challenge the psycho-oncology clinician to distinguish between normative and maladaptive responses.

A range of emotions, cognitions, behaviors, and physical symptoms characterizes adaptive grief.[3] These include:

Emotions
* sadness, anger, despair, anxiety, a predominant yearning for the deceased
* caregiver guilt and regret about choices made throughout the patient's illness and at the end of life
* distress and anguish regarding the patient's suffering
* relief that the patient is no longer suffering or that the heaviness of caregiving has ceased

Cognitions
* intrusive, unwanted imagery and thoughts about the patient's illness and death
* attempts to understand the medical or psychological factors responsible for the death
* reflection on comforting memories that become more accessible across time

Behaviors
* avoidance of painful reminders of the loss
* seeking out reminders of the deceased
* approach to or withdrawal from social interactions, sometimes alternating between the two

Physical symptoms
* sleep disturbances and fatigue
* appetite and weight loss
* tension and restlessness
* tremors and somatic pain.

Distressing symptoms in all four domains commonly ameliorate with time. However, this improvement sometimes ironically results in feelings of betrayal of the patient and survivors' guilt, of which clinicians should be mindful.

Adaptation to loss is commonly believed to follow the dual process model of coping,[9] with an oscillation between confronting the loss and related stressors, processing related emotions, and coping with the stressors of reengagement in and restoring life without the deceased physically present. The intensity and duration of grieving are significantly related to the strength and degree of attachment security. Though no evidence-based timelines for adaptation have been established, cultural norms and values may influence the duration and variant expressions of grief.

✔ Tool

Clinicians may consider illustrating the Dual Process Model of Coping by sketching this classic figure,[9] demonstrating the two spheres of stressors, loss- and restoration-focus, highlighting how it is typical and adaptive to oscillate between both domains. Explain that there may be a lack of predictability in a given day or week, but over time the broader pattern reflects the importance of coping with both the pain of loss and efforts to reengage in life without the deceased physically present.

✎ Checklist

Grief experiences are highly nuanced, but there are several indicators that an individual is beginning to adapt to loss, such as:
- Being able to acknowledge the reality of loss
- Transforming the relationship to the deceased into one that includes this new reality while maintaining a sense of connection

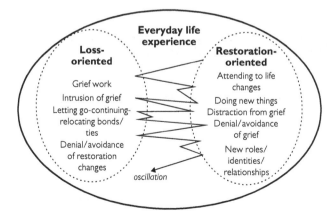

Figure 10.1 The Dual Process Model of Coping in Bereavement, adapted with permission from Stroebe M, Schut H. Death Studies, 1999; 23:197–224. https://www.uu.nl/staff/MSStroebe

- Developing or maintaining other personal relationships
- Re-engaging in work, leisure, and creative endeavors
- Being able to consider their lives and the future as potentially meaningful and satisfying

While it is expected that grief continues throughout an individual's life, reactions typically become less intense and briefer over time, with an increased ability to reminisce about their deceased loved one with emotional and mental equanimity. Resilience following significant loss is common, and it is expected that the vast majority of individuals (80%–90%) will cultivate ways to adapt to their loss. That said, it is important for clinicians to be aware that many grieving individuals may appear to be adapting but continue to struggle to some extent with navigating relationships and responsibilities.

Diagnosis and Assessment of Bereavement-Related Mental Health Challenges

Intense waves of sadness and anxiety are common and to be expected in the acute grief phase. For some individuals, however, the stress of bereavement may compound existing vulnerabilities, leading to pervasive, persistent depressed mood, or worsening of premorbid psychiatric conditions (see Box 10.2).

Anxiety is common among the bereaved as they reflect on a future without the deceased physically present. Some will meet criteria for *anxiety disorders*, presenting with symptoms of separation anxiety, panic disorder, generalized anxiety, and/or phobias. Symptoms of PTSD may emerge when circumstances of the death are perceived as traumatic, such as when the bereaved have witnessed the patient with gross disfigurement, open bedsores, or severe difficulty breathing; or when they learn about the patient's actual or threatened death. *Identification pain*, that is, pain in an area of the body that the patient experienced, can manifest, as can frank *somatization disorders*. In addition, those who have a history of *substance use, bipolar, or psychotic disorders* are at heightened risk of relapse as they face the stress of grief and

---

Box 10.2 Recognizing Clinical Depression among the Bereaved

- The Diagnostic and Statistical Manual for Mental Disorders, 5th Edition (DSM-5) allows for a diagnosis of depression if pertinent symptoms have been present and become pervasive for at least two weeks after experiencing the loss of a loved one.
- Considering that waves of sadness are so frequent during the early months of bereavement, clinicians should only make such a diagnosis during the acute stages of bereavement after carefully considering an individual's history and cultural norms regarding bereavement.
- The sadness that commonly accompanies a significant loss or reflections about a patient's suffering alone does not constitute a clinical depression.
- Major depression may occur more often among the newly bereaved who have a past or family history of clinical depression.

the related loss of active social support from the deceased. While aspects of adjustment disorder diagnoses commonly appear fitting for the bereaved, according to the rules of DSM-5, these diagnoses should be deferred if the clinical symptoms are related to normal bereavement.

Prolonged Grief Disorder

Prolonged grief disorder (PGD)—formerly referred to as both complicated grief and traumatic grief—is characterized by a more protracted and severe grief response without abatement over time and occurs in approximately 8% of grieving caregivers.[2,10] PGD has been established as a distinct mental disorder in the International Classification of Diseases-11 (ICD-11) and requires the following criteria for diagnosis:

- Death of a close person
- Persistent and pervasive grief response accompanied by longing for or pre-occupation with deceased
- Intense emotional pain (sadness, guilt, anger, denial, blame, lost sense of self, absence of positive mood, numbness, avoidance of social and other activities)
- Minimum of 6 months after death, exceeding social, cultural, and religious norms
- Significant impairment in personal, family, social, occupational, or other functioning.

Prigerson et al. detailed the most recent criteria for the disorder included in the DSM-5-Text Revision (DSM-5-TR),[10] which state that the diagnosis should not be made until at least 12 months have elapsed since the death. This duration was selected to identify individuals whose grief is persistent and who may benefit from intervention, while not being overly inclusive of individuals exhibiting more typical grief reactions.

Individuals with PGD may appear "stuck" in their grief, intensely pining and yearning for the lost individual. They may experience distressing ruminations and intrusive thoughts about the absence of the deceased, a struggle to find meaning in their lives without their loved one, and difficulty accepting the reality of the loss and engaging in life.[10] Symptoms of PGD have been empirically distinguished from symptoms of anxiety or depression (e.g., depressed mood, changes in appetite or weight).[10] PGD may be a consequence of either traumatic or nontraumatic losses and has been associated with increased risk of negative mental and physical health outcomes, including cancer, hypertension, cardiac events, adverse health behaviors, and suicidal ideation.[10]

Assessment and Bereavement Risk Factors

The majority of individuals who experience a loss will gradually adapt without need for psychosocial interventions. However, a subset of individuals is at risk for poor outcomes in bereavement, such as those described above.[8] Neimeyer and Burke[7] categorized prospective, empirically validated risk factors of PGD as:

- Background (e.g., dependency on the deceased, multiple loss)
- Illness/treatment-related impact (e.g., witnessing intensive medical interventions, perceiving the death as traumatic)
- Death/bereavement-related (e.g., regret, isolation)

Other risk factors include being a spouse or parent of the deceased, having low social support, high levels of neuroticism, insecure attachment styles, history of trauma or mental health problems, or a history of separation anxiety.[7,8,11] See Table 10.2.

When bereavement resources are limited, as they often are, it can be helpful to identify those at greater risk for maladaptive coping so they can be referred for professional support in a timely manner. Holding a regular multi-disciplinary death review can facilitate identification of family members at risk for psychopathology.[12]

Table 10.2 Risk Factors of Poor Bereavement Outcomes

Risk Factor	Empirical Findings
Circumstances of death	Violent, sudden, traumatic deaths; distressing circumstances such as uncontrolled pain, difficulty breathing, delirium, or being alone
Demographic characteristics of the bereaved	Women at higher risk than men;* those with financial hardship and/or lower education
Relationship to the deceased	First-degree relatives, with parents and spouses at highest risk
Social support	Low social support and isolation
Family functioning	Low cohesion and communication, and high conflict
Attachment style	Insecure attachment styles, particularly anxious attachment styles
Meaning-making	Challenges with meaning-making, particularly sense-making
Dependency on the deceased	Increased emotional and practical dependency, particularly among spouses/partners
Mental health or trauma history	History of mental health challenges, including separation anxiety, or traumatic experiences
Caregiver experiences	Increased caregiver burden; greater length and intensity of caregiving
Pre-death grief and preparation for the loss	Higher levels of anticipatory and illness-related grief, decreased preparedness for the loss
Unresolved relational issues with the deceased	Preoccupying levels of guilt, regret, and/or unfinished business or history of conflict with the deceased
Loss history	Early traumatic loss and (all lower case) multiple losses, especially in quick succession (bereavement overload)
Institutional circumstances	Lack of support, disengagement of family from caregiving at the end of life, or inadequate communication with medical staff in care settings

Note. Adapted from Neimeyer[8] and Lichtenthal et al.[16]
* Researchers may have historically limited survey questions to binary gender identity options.

⚲ Key Message

Bereavement risk screening should be conducted prior to family members experiencing a loss to more effectively triage outreach efforts to those most in need of support and to connect family members to services pre-loss to prevent them from "falling through the cracks."[11] Individuals at highest risk can be linked to professional support, which may prevent the development of mental and physical health morbidity in bereavement.[11]

Specific Loss Circumstances for Consideration

Sudden Death. Despite the protracted nature of many cancers, deaths may be perceived as unexpected or sudden by family members because they often expect or hope for more time with the patient. Unexpected deaths can also result from secondary conditions related to illness, treatment, or hospitalization complications (e.g., sepsis, pulmonary emboli, cardiac events, hemorrhage). Individuals who perceive themselves as psychologically unprepared for the loss are at greater risk for PGD and depression, particularly when the death is perceived as traumatic.[7] Clinicians should assess family members' understanding of the circumstances surrounding the death and assist the bereaved in making sense of any aspects that were perplexing.

Childhood Grief. Children's developmental stage directly informs their ability to comprehend the permanence of death and to express their grief. Clinicians should consider that the capacity for abstract thinking develops around ages 8–10. Transparent, age-appropriate discussion of the loss accompanied by support from surviving family members promotes adaptive grieving for children. Suggestions to support the adaptive process include participation in mourning rituals, facilitation of emotional expression through, for example, physical activities, and creation of a memory book to preserve the child's bond to the deceased. Professional evaluation and intervention may be called for if intense, impairing grief reactions persist beyond six months. A holistic and child-centered approach should be integrated into bereavement care.

Loss of a Child. Parents who suffer the death of a child often have profound grief reactions.[13,14] Like many adults with cancer, losing a child often follows a lengthy battle with illness. When caregiving for their child has been the top priority for so long, parents may become disconnected from relationships and roles that were previously meaningful. The severe pain of acute grief may intensify the sense of isolation. They may feel estranged from the clinicians who treated their child, complicating bereavement follow-up through which referrals for additional support can be offered as a standard of care.[14] Parents may find comfort engaging with other bereaved parents through support groups, both onsite and online. They may also require assistance coping with any guilt related to doubts that they could or should have done more to prevent the death. Clinicians can explore ways to honor and memorialize the child's life. Parents may use memories of their child in their daily life to learn to co-exist with their grief.[13]

COVID-19. The COVID-19 pandemic has complicated palliative care provision and bereavement for many family members and caregivers worldwide.[15,16] Visitor restriction policies, pervasive fear of viral transmission, disconnection from spiritual support communities, social distancing mandates, and limitations on public gatherings have all interacted to interrupt the normal grieving process and further disenfranchise grief for already marginalized populations and higher bereavement risk groups (e.g., parents suffering the loss of a child).[15,16] Cancer patients were more vulnerable to the virus; many died whose cancer itself was not expected to take their lives at the time of their deaths, leaving families struggling with making sense of their loss. Furthermore, support has been generally compromised. Clinicians should be mindful that the impact of these circumstances on grievers may be long-lasting, even for mourners whose loved ones died of other causes during the pandemic, but who suffered from many of the same contextual risk factors as those who died of COVID-19.[15,16]

Stigmatized deaths. In some countries, *death from physician-assisted suicide* and *euthanasia* has become stigmatized. Like other commonly stigmatized deaths (e.g., suicides, homicides, accidental drug overdoses), stigma can result in shame and embarrassment, hindering family members from sharing the cause of death with others. This can impede discussion about the loss and therefore opportunities for emotional processing and social support. Family members may also experience anger at the deceased over their choice of death and the suddenness with which the death occurred, leaving them feeling shortchanged in the end. Religious communities may create further discomfort. In locations where physician-assisted suicide has been legalized, there have been efforts to organize special bereavement services to accommodate the needs of surviving family members.

Differential Diagnosis

Because acute grief is typically distressing, particularly in the immediate wake of a loss, differential diagnosis between this common response and bereavement-related mental disorders is essential.

✔ Tool
Clinicians should consider:
• *the timing of the symptoms*
• *their persistence*
• *their intensity, and*
• *whether they are impairing functioning.*

With typical grief, symptoms are usually most intense within the first year after a significant loss. Emotions commonly come in waves. Over time, the intensity tends to diminish, with resurgences around reminders of the deceased's absence, the death anniversary, holidays, and milestones. Grief is never expected to resolve completely; throughout a bereaved individual's life, there may always be circumstances that will trigger waves of grief.

When acute grief symptoms persist and result in impairment or elevated distress, a PGD diagnosis may be considered. As noted previously, PGD does not equate only to continued yearning for the deceased, but rather is defined by the presence of multiple intense and persistent symptoms such as meaninglessness, identity challenges, and anger, and functional debilitation.[10] Clinicians must take into account contextual factors and should be cautious about pathologizing grief responses. PGD can be distinguished from other mental health challenges such as MDD and PTSD by its focus on separation distress and the lost relationship. PGD symptoms tend to be more stable than those of MDD. Among grieving individuals with MDD, sadness is more pervasive, and negative thoughts focus more on the self, the world, and the future rather than on the deceased.

Cognitions among those experiencing PTSD commonly focus on events during the patient's illness or circumstances of death. Individuals with PTSD commonly avoid reminders of the traumatic circumstances, fearing reliving them and related disturbing imagery, whereas those with PGD may avoid reminders of the deceased's absence, longing for reunion with the deceased. In fact, bereaved individuals suffering from PGD may deliberately reminisce about the deceased, whereas individuals with PTSD typically avoid thinking about the traumatic experience. This said, individuals may experience comorbid conditions, including PTSD, PGD, and/or MDD, and clinicians will need to walk a fine line between distinguishing mental health disorders in bereavement and considering that some bereaved individuals may be suffering from multiple mental health disorders in the wake of their loss.

Clinical Management

Before and around the Patient's Death

Empathic communication is critical to helping families process important information and cope as the patient's illness progresses. As families adapt to numerous losses in the context of serious illness and express their attachment through caregiving, they may grow closer and more cohesive.[12] Psycho-oncology clinicians should promote transparent communication and opportunities to say goodbye. They can also encourage patients and families to resolve unfinished business, express appreciation for each other, and address relationship issues when possible.[12] Families exhibiting greater dysfunction may struggle with communication and medical decision-making, particularly at the end of the patient's life and when patients are unable to communicate.[6] Anticipatory grief may challenge surrogate decision-makers to consistently make choices aligned with the patient's values, increasing their risk for bereavement adjustment difficulties.[6,12] Some members may react with denial, hostility, intense anxiety, avoidance, or other maladaptive behaviors, resulting in tension and conflict.[12]

Psycho-oncology clinicians must demonstrate the highest possible respect and sensitivity for the fragility of the unfolding human experience during this period. Practitioners' therapeutic presence and empathic communication can offer vital reassurance regarding the patient's comfort, in addition to providing necessary information about the dying process (e.g., meaning of sounds, changes of breathing patterns and levels of consciousness). Providing a safe space for consideration of the patient's and family's values and the tensions between life-prolonging and palliative care may help mitigate regret.

Acting as bereavement-conscious clinicians,[3] staff should contact family members or designated surrogates who are unable to be present when the patient's condition begins to deteriorate and death appears imminent. If the death occurs prior to family arrival, they should be offered an opportunity to view the body after it has been cleaned, cared for, and invasive medical devices have been removed (with the exception of patients who will likely bleed heavily or those awaiting autopsy). Family members should be given information about the sequence of events leading up to the death. Staff must integrate cultural and religious needs into the delivery of care, including desires related to autopsy, time alone with the patient, and pastoral counseling. Involving religious and/or cultural communities and leaders as requested by family members may provide an extra layer of psychosocial and spiritual support. Culture and cultural norms influence how family members express acute grief, and clinicians could consult with a cultural intermediary to ensure their response is sensitive to needs. Expected deaths should not be minimized in an effort to prevent disenfranchised grief. Clinicians may consider prescribing anxiolytics or sleep aids, guidance on funeral arrangements, and referrals for specialized bereavement services.

Following the Patient's Death

Condolence calls. Families have expressed that continuity of care through phone calls, letters, or other personal means is greatly appreciated after the patient's death.[14] Clinicians' efforts to follow up with bereaved families after the patient's death, expressing their condolences by telephone, sympathy card, or personal visits, by funeral attendance, or through annual commemoration services are generally welcome.[16] These calls can include expressions of sadness, personal reflections about and appreciation for the patient, and amplification of the fact that their lives "mattered." They can also include a risk assessment and referrals for care when family members appear to be at higher risk or indicate an interest in continued support.[16]

Ongoing Support. Psychosocial care of the family following the patient's death can prevent feelings of abandonment that some family members have reported when they experience a sudden disconnection from providers after the patient's death.[14] In encounters with bereaved family members, it is vital that psycho-oncology clinicians emphasize the broad range of psychosocial and physical challenges commonly faced by the bereaved in the wake of loss. When grieving persons think they "should be" reacting differently than they are, it can exacerbate their distress and negatively affect adaptation to the loss. Family members reviewing their behaviors and experiencing related guilt and regret should be reminded that such feelings are common and that, in most cases, there is no "right" or "wrong." Psychoeducation about theories of coping (see Table 10.1) can help survivors make sense of the fluctuations of their reactions and needs.

⚹ Key Message

Much of what clinicians offer in response to acute grief is psychoeducation about common responses to loss and encouragement to give themselves permission to grieve. Clinicians can normalize the unpredictability of their feelings and support them in learning to surf the waves of emotions that come and go.

Specific Psychosocial Grief Interventions

Most bereaved individuals (~ 80%–90%) do not require specific interventions because their symptoms dissipate naturally over time, though some may still find supportive grief counseling valuable. For individuals presenting with more clinical symptomatology, specific grief therapy approaches may be warranted.

Supportive Counseling

Several supportive grief therapy techniques can assist clinicians in holistically supporting grieving family members in an adaptive grieving process, including normalization, validation, and facilitation of emotional processing. Supportive counseling can provide a safe and protected space to speak about the deceased and express emotions without concerns about family members' and friends' reactions, which commonly impacts what bereaved individuals share with others. It can also offer a forum to organically engage in meaning-making and to reflect on how to reengage in life without the deceased physically present.[8] Supportive elements are key in a variety of more specific grief intervention approaches, though purely supportive counseling may be less effective in reducing PGD symptoms than cognitive-behavioral interventions.[4]

Meaning-Focused Psychotherapies

These therapies incorporate constructivist and existential approaches and are commonly used with grieving populations. Specifically, meaning reconstruction can help bereaved individuals find meaning in their loss, facilitating development of a narrative about the lost relationship and the loss event.[8] It focuses on the challenges to meaning-making that the loss has resulted in, such as invalidating assumptions about the way life works, the meaning of their ongoing bond with the deceased, and the significance of their own life as a bereaved person. The therapist helps the griever to process the event story of the death through approaches such as narrative retelling and directed journaling, to access the back story of the relationship to the deceased through exercises such as imaginal conversations and letter writing, and to revise their own sense of identity accordingly.[8]

Meaning-Centered Grief Therapy (MCGT) is a 16-session manualized intervention developed by our group that incorporates meaning reconstruction to help the bereaved re-author adaptive narratives about their loss and their lives.[13] It further assists the bereaved in the existential pursuit of meaning by facilitating their connection to sources of meaning, which help them coexist with their continued grief.

- Sessions 1 and 2 provide psychoeducation about the core concepts of MCGT, prolonged grief reactions, and experiential avoidance, eliciting an understanding of beliefs about grief and emotions, and encouraging the bereaved to identify a way to making meaning of their emotional reactions with compassion. They invite deliberate connection to the deceased.

- In Session 3 and 4, connection to the deceased is deepened through review of the deceased's living legacy and how it is interwoven with the griever's story, which they may narrate however they choose.
- In Session 5, challenges to the mourner's sense of identity are explored.
- In Sessions 6 to 8, the therapist invites discussion of the griever's story as a source of meaning, reflecting on influences of the past, sources of meaning in the present, and inviting reflection on the ingredients of a meaningful future.
- In Session 9, during which a support provider is invited to join, barriers to meaningful connections are given attention.
- Sessions 10 to 12 explore other key sources of meaning, including choosing one's attitude in the face of limitations and pain, the way we engage in life, and connecting experiences.
- Sessions 13 and 14 revisit how the griever makes meaning of their loss experience, focusing on the most emotional components and finding a greater significance in the adversity they have faced.
- Sessions 15 and 16 conclude with amplifying the deceased's living legacy through a project the griever creates, and the ways they have chosen to find meaning in their life and loss as they look to the future. MCGT has demonstrated promise in reducing PGD and depressive symptoms in parents bereaved by cancer.[13] Recent extensions of a meaning-oriented model also draw on evidence-based procedures to promote co-construction of meaning in the family context.[17]

Psychodynamic and Interpersonal Psychotherapies

Psychodynamic approaches focus on the influence of childhood events, unconscious conflicts, and internalized patterns of relating to others that are reenacted in adult life and may influence the bereaved individual's grief reactions. Individuals who struggle with unresolved issues influenced by early relationships and conflicts, including those related to attachment security, might benefit from a psychodynamic approach, which is typically longer-term. Interpersonal psychotherapy (IPT) is a time-limited (12–16 weeks) manualized intervention, which is based partly on psychodynamic theory, and focuses on complicated grief when relevant for the bereaved individual. With its focus on relationship problems, IPT is indicated for those who are facing challenges with interpersonal functioning.

Cognitive-Behavioral Therapy (CBT)

CBT approaches with bereaved individuals focus on addressing maladaptive thoughts and behaviors that may play a role in persistent, debilitating grief. Cognitions related to guilt, regret, anger, and coping with distress and the future may be targeted. Exposure exercises to reduce avoidance of distressing feelings, thoughts, and behaviors may be especially helpful.[4] Such exercises may assist grievers with reengaging in restorative activities. Behavioral activation, which involves identifying behavioral goals and engaging in pleasurable activities, may be particularly useful for bereaved older adults.[18] CBT has demonstrated efficacy in reducing PGD as compared to supportive counseling, and there is evidence suggesting that including exposure techniques results in greater reductions of PGD symptoms than using cognitive techniques alone.[4] Third-wave CBT approaches that address how an individual relates to thoughts and emotions, incorporating concepts such as mindfulness, metacognition, and acceptance, are increasingly being incorporated into grief interventions and may be used in conjunction with traditional CBT approaches.

Prolonged Grief Disorder Treatment (PGDT)

Developed and rigorously researched by Shear and colleagues,[19] PGDT is an individual intervention developed specifically to treat PGD. PGDT is a 16-session manualized treatment that applies CBT and IPT principles and includes psychoeducation about the dual process model of coping, exposure to avoided loss-related thoughts, retelling the story of the death, imaginal conversations with the deceased, and development of personal goals to assist with restorative behaviors. Research has suggested PGDT is more efficacious and quicker in reducing PGD symptoms than IPT.[19]

Group Psychotherapy

The mutual support and validation offered by those who have experienced similar losses is a primary benefit of group-based grief interventions. Groups may also reduce bereaved individuals' sense of isolation, promote emotional expression and processing, and offer an opportunity for group members to share effective coping strategies with one another. Clinicians can use a group format to deliver general supportive counseling or more specific psychotherapeutic approaches, such as CBT, tailored for bereaved populations.

Family Therapy

The routine use of family-oriented screening and family-centered intervention may be invaluable in supporting high-risk families in oncology settings.[12] For example, Kissane and colleagues[12] developed Family-Focused Grief Therapy (FFGT) to foster care continuity through a 6 to 10 session preventive intervention for high-risk families that commences during palliative care with the patient and continues with surviving family members after the patient's death. Families are screened to identify relevant risk factors associated with negative bereavement outcomes, including high conflict, low cohesion, and/or communication deficits. Dysfunctional and "at risk" families displaying moderate levels of disturbance are targeted.[12] FFGT addresses families' risk factors by fostering open communication, promoting mutual support and the sharing of grief. An RCT comparing 10 sessions of FFGT to standard care for low-communication and high-conflict families compared to low-involvement families found lower rates of PGD in those who received FFGT compared to the control group.[12]

Online Intervention

The delivery of Internet-based grief interventions may be especially valuable for the bereft who cannot easily access support or who find it emotionally challenging to return to the institution where the patient was treated. Individual and group online formats have been described in recent reviews.[4,18] The majority of studies have tested CBT approaches, which have demonstrated promise in improving a number of mental health outcomes, such as depression and PTSD symptoms.[4,18] Interestingly, online interventions have demonstrated efficacy regardless of age group, including older adults.

Psychopharmacological Approaches
Bereavement-related mental disorders are often treated using standard psychopharmacological and psychotherapeutic approaches.

ꓘ Checklist

- Anxiolytics and sleep aids may be particularly useful during the acute phase of bereavement.
- Among those who exhibit clinical levels of depression, selective serotonin reuptake inhibitors (SSRIs) and selective noradrenergic reuptake inhibitors (SNRIs) may be used to reduce depressive symptoms.
- For severe and debilitating symptoms of PGD, pharmacological treatments may be indicated. Although evidence in this domain remains extremely limited, a number of medications have been trialed, including SSRIs and benzodiazepines.
- SSRIs have shown only moderate effectiveness in mitigating grief symptoms, albeit in the setting of methodological concerns (e.g., lack of randomization and blinding, small sample size, comorbid mental health disorders).[20]
- The time lag to achieve full efficacy for SSRIs (e.g., weeks to months) should also be considered alongside the severity of grief symptoms.
- Tricyclic antidepressants (TCAs) and benzodiazepines have not been shown as effective psychopharmacological interventions for PGD symptom reduction.[20]

Professional Issues and Service Implementation

Recording and Communicating Challenges

Disenfranchised groups may harbor distrust of the health system or of clinicians, and thus building trust is key to ensuring quality bereavement care. Cultural sensitivity and inclusive, empathic communication practices should be utilized consistently for both patients and their social support systems (e.g., caregivers, families of origin, families of choice). Instances where there has been inconsistent support, trust, or relationship-building between clinicians and care recipients may pose challenges to effective communication.

Psycho-oncology clinicians may need to use creative approaches to communicating with interdisciplinary colleagues across care teams to strategize bereavement care, given resources and clinical priorities. Regular multidisciplinary meetings to identify high-risk family members can be invaluable to ensuring the appropriate level of bereavement care prior to the patient's death. Coordination of bereavement outreach, including condolence calls and messages, can ensure that no family member falls through the cracks. The documentation of such efforts can be complicated, however, when family members do not have their own medical records, adding notes about family communication in the deceased patient's records can infringe on privacy and impede appropriate follow-up when the family is in clinical need.[21] Creating a separate medical record for the family member is optimal whenever possible.[21]

Legal Responsibilities

Psycho-oncology clinicians should convey empathy for the legal challenges that bereaved family members often confront, such as the managing of the deceased's estate. They should employ ethical consultation practices and social work support as needed for families that become fractured over estate disagreements. They should communicate sensitively when declining to witness wills or participate in legal paperwork completion beyond their scope of practice.

Common Ethical Dilemmas

Physician-assisted suicide (PAS) deaths and euthanasia have unique impacts on bereavement that require a nonjudgmental therapeutic presence for surviving caregivers, who may be struggling with the end of life decisions of the deceased. PAS may further exacerbate moral distress, which is the result of clinicians believing there is a "right" clinical action to take that aligns with their own moral compass but being unable to act accordingly due to systemic constraints. Reports of moral distress and moral suffering have also risen throughout the COVID-19 pandemic. Clinicians should be aware of their own transference in these situations and seek out mental health supports as needed. In instances where medical errors have resulted in death, psycho-oncology clinicians should acknowledge their impact on the bereaved, while considering their dual loyalties to their employers' legal position and their own individual ethical code of professional conduct.

Policies for Clinical Services

Bereavement care services need to be addressed appropriately. All levels of health systems require funding and investment to develop and staff programs. Palliative care and psycho-oncology curricula and training programs should be expanded to include an adequate focus on bereavement care and to support the development of bereavement-conscious clinicians.[3] Policies that promote diversity, equity, and inclusion for disenfranchised groups and individuals are needed to address the historic marginalization of minoritized groups, and ensure relationship-based bereavement care that recognizes the social contexts of families and communities. Culturally sensitive policies are needed at institutional levels to ensure bereavement care is reflective of cultural norms and values, and to invest in community-based partnerships with cultural groups to build respectful relationships with those being served.

Teams and Supervision Challenges

An important consideration in every psycho-oncologists' practice is professional grief, as clinicians face the death of patients with whom they have developed close connections (see Chapter 11), as well as the cumulative loss of patients over time.[22] The marked increase of loss and grief confronted by health professionals during the COVID-19 pandemic has heightened endorsement of anxiety, PTSD, helplessness and isolation among various groups of professionals. Long before the pandemic, health professionals suffered high levels of burnout, an occupational phenomenon characterized by poor work environments and job responsibilities that outweigh available resources, including time to invest in bereavement care. Interventions are needed to support health professionals as they grieve. Both individual coping strategies (e.g., seeking social support, problem solving, applying meaning-centered strategies) and workplace measures (e.g., coaching, staff support and recognition, clear communication, holding patient memorials) may be helpful in promoting health professionals' psychological well-being.[22]

Interventions are needed to support health professionals who are coping with grief over losses of patients and colleagues.[22] Meaning-centered therapeutic care, designed to address existential and emotional burdens of patients with cancer, may be adapted to meet the needs of health professionals. In the context of the pandemic, a coaching approach to staff debriefing delivered in an empathic manner may create work cultures that can mitigate the unprecedented distress of the global workforce.[22]

Implementation Considerations

🔑 Key Message

The psycho-oncologist delivering palliative care is ultimately seeking to alleviate suffering and enhance quality of life for the person confronting serious illness and the family members and caregivers who support them. Although bereavement care is often an afterthought in many acute care settings or during disease-directed treatment, clinicians should consistently plan and deliver services with both anticipatory grief and bereavement concerns in mind.[3]

There are several major challenges to optimizing bereavement care in psycho-oncology. The first is that few professionals working in oncology have received even minimal training in bereavement care, even within palliative care specialist settings. The second is that resources—including dedicated time and staff—for bereavement support are quite limited in cancer care. Resource constraints have only become more severe in the wake of the COVID-19 pandemic, further limiting the physical and emotional capacity of psycho-oncologists. Guidelines for bereavement care have been proposed but not routinely implemented.[23] Interdisciplinary collaboration is key to effectively and sustainably leverage a team approach to implement family-centered bereavement care where the prevalence of loss is high. Each team should identify which team member has the capacity and skills needed to make follow-up contact with the bereaved in due time. Psycho-oncologists can play a key role in translating bereavement care recommendations into practice.

References

1. Wright AA, Zhang B, Ray A, et al. Associations between end of life discussions, patient mental health, medical care near death, and caregiver bereavement adjustment. JAMA.2008;300:1665–1673.

2. Nielsen MK, Neergaard MA, Jensen AB, et al. Predictors of complicated grief and depression in bereaved caregivers: A nationwide prospective cohort study. J Pain Symptom Manage. 2017;53:540–550.

3. Roberts KE, Lichtenthal WG, Ferrell BR. Being a bereavement-conscious hospice and palliative care clinician. J Hosp and Palliat Nursing. 2021;23:293–295.

4. Johannsen M, Damholdt MF, Zachariae R, et al. Psychological interventions for grief in adults: A systematic review and meta-analysis of randomized controlled trials. J Affect Disord. 2019;253:69–86.

5. Singer J, Roberts KE, McLean E, et al. An examination of family members grief prior to loss of individuals with a life limiting illness: A systematic review. Under review. (Update at proof stage).

6. Lichtenthal WG, Viola M, Rogers M, et al. Development and preliminary evaluation of EMPOWER for surrogate decision-makers of critically ill patients. Palliat Support Care. 2021:1–11.

7. Neimeyer RA, Burke LA. What makes grief complicated? Risk factors for complicated grief. In Doka K, Tucci A, Editors. Living with Grief: When Grief Is Complicated. Hospice Washington, DC: Foundation of America; 2017. Pages 73–93.

8. Neimeyer RA. Meaning reconstruction in bereavement: Development of a research program. Death Stud. 2019;43:79–91.

9. Stroebe M, Schut H. The dual process model of coping with bereavement: Rationale and description. Death Stud. 1999;23:197–224.

10. Prigerson HG, Boelen PA, Xu J, et al. Validation of the new DSM-5-TR criteria for prolonged grief disorder and the PG-13-Revised (PG-13-R) scale. World Psychiatry. 2021;20:96–106.

11. Roberts KE, Jankauskaite G, Slivjak E, et al. Bereavement risk screening: A pathway to psychosocial oncology care. Psycho-Oncology. 2020;29:2041–2047.

12. Kissane DW, Zaider TI, Li Y, et al. Randomized controlled trial of family therapy in advanced cancer continued into bereavement. J Clin Oncol. 2016;34:1921–1927.

13. Lichtenthal WG, Catarozoli C, Masterson M, et al. An open trial of Meaning-Centered Grief Therapy: Rationale and preliminary evaluation. Palliat Support Care. 2019;17:2–12.

14. Lichtenthal WG, Sweeney CR, Roberts KE, et al. Bereavement follow-up after the death of a child as a standard of care in pediatric oncology. Pediatr Blood Cancer. 2015;62 Suppl 5:S834–869.

15. Neimeyer RA, Lee SA. Circumstances of the death and associated risk factors for severity and impairment of COVID-19 grief. Death Stud. 2021:1–9.

16. Lichtenthal WG, Roberts KE, Prigerson HG. Bereavement care in the wake of COVID-19: Offering condolences and referrals. Ann Intern Med 2020;173:833–835.

17. Barboza J, Seedall R, Neimeyer RA: Meaning co-construction: Facilitating shared family meaning-making in bereavement. Fam Process. 2021. (Update at proof stage)

18. Roberts KE, Walsh LE, Saracino RM, Fogarty J, Coats T, Goldberg J, Prigerson H, Lichtenthal WG. A systematic review of treatment options for grieving older adults. Curr Treat Opt Psychiatry. 2019;6:422–449.

19. Shear MK, Reynolds CF 3rd, Simon NM, et al. Optimizing treatment of complicated grief: A randomized clinical trial. JAMA Psychiatry. 2016;73:685–694.

20. Bui E, Nadal-Vicens M, Simon NM. Pharmacological approaches to the treatment of complicated grief: Rationale and a brief review of the literature. Dialogues Clin Neurosci. 2012;14:149–157.

21. Applebaum AJ, Kent EE, Lichtenthal WG. Documentation of caregivers as a standard of care. J Clin Oncol. 2021;39:1955–1958.

22. Rosa WE, Levoy K, Battista V, et al. Using the nurse coaching process to support bereaved staff during the COVID-19 crisis. J Hosp Palliat Nurs. 2021;23:403–405.

23. Hudson P, Hall C, Boughey A, et al. Bereavement support standards and bereavement care pathway for quality palliative care. Palliat Support Care. 2018;16:375–387.

Further Reading

Kissane DW, Parnes F, Editors. Bereavement Care for Families. New York: Routledge; 2014. A practical, multiauthored guide to bereavement care using family approaches.

Neimeyer, RA, Editor. New Techniques of Grief Therapy: Bereavement and Beyond. New York: Routledge; 2022. Novel and worthwhile techniques to support the bereaved.

Neimeyer RA. Techniques of Grief Therapy: Creative Practices for Counseling the Bereaved. New York: Routledge; 2012. Clinically useful guide of intervention approaches to incorporate into grief therapy.

Waller A, Turon H, Mansfield E, et al. Assisting the bereaved: A systematic review of the evidence for grief counselling. Palliat Med. 2016;30:132–148. An overview of studies of grief interventions.

Worden JW. Grief Counseling and Grief Therapy: A Handbook for the Mental Health Practitioner. 5th ed. New York: Springer Publishing Company; 2018. Classic tome on grief therapy.

Chapter 11

Staff Support

Brian Kelly, Maria Die Trill, and Christian Ntizimira

Learning Objectives

After reading this chapter the clinician will be able to:

1. Describe the common psychological responses experienced by clinicians providing end of life care.
2. Outline both risk and protective factors that influence the impact of end of life care on clinicians.
3. Describe commonly used strategies at both organizational and individual levels that can improve psychological outcomes for clinicians.
4. Describe the role of cultural (including spiritual) factors relevant to the support of palliative care providers.
5. Outline examples of models of palliative care relevant to diverse cultural and geographic settings, and the role of caregiver support and education in the provision of such models of care.

Background Evidence

Palliative care can be a demanding specialty that requires continued contact with severely ill patients in situations of physical and psychological deterioration and suffering. Caring for patients facing the end of life and their families can also be rewarding in many ways. Now, more than ever, palliative care specialists confront multiple challenges that may place them at risk for developing physical, emotional, spiritual, and psychological distress, possibly limiting their ability to provide compassionate care.[1]

The well-being of clinicians is considered one of the key goals of healthcare, along with improving population health, containment of cost, and improving patient experience.[2] While the potential impact on clinicians of working in palliative care is readily acknowledged and understood, this is also balanced by the sense of achievement and personal rewards in such work.

Helping patients find meaning in suffering, helping them and their relatives navigate throughout the dying process, learning to appreciate one's own life as a gift, and an increased awareness of one's spirituality are gains from working in this field. In addition, daily spiritual practices mitigate the physical, cognitive, and emotional forms of burnout that may develop.

High levels of stress may lead to so-called "burnout" responses, which include emotional exhaustion, depersonalization, and a sense of reduced personal accomplishment. A systematic literature review revealed that rates of burnout in palliative care clinicians varies widely (3% to 66%).[3] No major differences in prevalence were found between nurses and physicians. Healthcare professionals providing palliative care in a general health setting experienced more symptoms of burnout than those in specialized palliative care settings.

Staff caring for patients at the end of life are subject to their own grief responses. These losses need to be efficiently worked through in order to provide optimal care while avoiding emotional detachment from patients. Staff grief is not usually recognized. Disenfranchised grief appears when grief is hidden and grief reactions are not expressed.[4]

Compassion fatigue refers to "cynicism, emotional exhaustion or self-centeredness occuring in a healthcare professional previously dedicated to his/her work with patients." [5] It is a form of exhaustion resulting from prolonged exposure to caring for sick or traumatized patients. Compassion fatigue affects the healthcare staff´s job satisfaction as well as patient outcomes and may result in staff leaving their profession. The consequences of such compassion fatigue include the loss of ability to feel compassion and empathy, burnout, breakdown, disinterest, and moral distress.

The domains of compassion fatigue (see Table 11.1) can impact on many aspects of a clinician's life, and align closely with the common symptoms or signs of stress, which may arise among palliative care clinicians.

Table 11.1 Compassion Fatigue Domains[9]

EMOTIONAL AND PSYCHOLOGICAL	Palliative care staff may compartmentalize their feelings to avoid feeling the stress of multiple deaths[10] with diminished empathy, irritability and depersonalization of care
	Difficulty maintaining professional boundaries leading to role confusion
	Heightened sense of burden of patient care
	Sense of personal exhaustion
	Loss of sense of purpose or meaning in work, with feelings of demoralization
INTELLECTUAL AND PROFESSIONAL	Difficulty concentrating on work tasks and reduced job performance
	Increased team conflict and interpersonal tensions in the workplace
	Feeling overwhelmed by work demands
PHYSICAL	Poor self-care (lack of sleep; increased physical complaints; escalating use of alcohol to cope)
SOCIAL	Inability to share in suffering with others; difficulty enjoying outside life[10]
	Inability to "switch off" from work related concerns
SPIRITUAL	Spiritual disconnection; inability to provide judgment on a spiritual level[11]

The impact of death and dying in the palliative care context has been intensified during the COVID-19 pandemic. This context illustrates the clinical, ethical, and psychosocial complexity of end of life care, and provides relevant lessons to guide preparation for future needs in palliative care, for instance, when facing unanticipated new and emerging challenges to healthcare systems and services. In the midst of the current pandemic, palliative care specialists are confronted with added burdens that include being exposed to an increased number of deaths in sometimes uncontrolled, chaotic situations throughout the institution where they work. They have to take over the care of dying patients in non-palliative-care settings, where staff are not knowledgeable about death and dying issues. They need to maintain complex end of life discussions with patients and families around advanced directives and other delicate issues in the "coldness" of telemedicine, or while wearing personal protection equipment, and with important time restrictions. Lack of human and other resources, the isolation needs of patients who may deteriorate quickly, and staff exposure to the risk of being infected with the virus require that palliative care staff members be offered psychological support to deal with the COVID-19 experience. Palliative care staff can struggle to balance the need for closeness to patients at the end of life, and the emotional distance that prevents them from feeling overwhelmed by their work. Addressing one's own mortality, recognizing personal and professional limitations, questioning issues such as what took them to practice in the palliative care field, and being able to listen and respond to patients' demands, fears, and uncertainties are fundamental to achieve emotional stability when working with the dying.

🔍 Key Point

Cultural issues must be taken into account in palliative care, and may constitute an added burden for healthcare professionals. People confront illness, death, and dying in different ways in diverse cultural contexts. These can reflect the differing views about death, diverse cultural practices surrounding the care of the dying, differing culture-based family roles and social practices, expectations and beliefs about healthcare, and the extent to which healthcare is responsive to these cultural needs.

Palliative care volunteers are also highly influenced by their caregiving activity. Many volunteers become involved in hospice and palliative care because of their own experiences with family members and/or friends who have died. Most volunteers report that they have experienced changes in some way since they began volunteering (e.g., they have grown in some way, have learned how to keep things in perspective).

🔍 Key Point

Attention needs to be given to appropriate oversight, coordination, training, and support of volunteers to mitigate risks of personal burden and distress, especially when not protected by the structures of professional boundaries and roles that help manage emotional demands and workload.

From an international perspective, end of life care for many people occurs in less-resourced community settings, without the benefits of a broad-based multidisciplinary team, limited access to traditional specialist interventions, and care embedded within the community, with reliance on nonprofessional care providers. Nevertheless, models of care in these settings can provide insights into innovative methods to provide care that is appropriate to the cultural and resource context across diverse settings, and instructive examples of ways to support providers of community embedded end of life care.

Presenting Problems

Staff may develop some of the following:
- Workplace absences
- Clinical errors
- Reduced standards of practice
- Poorer communication
- Loss of compassion or empathy
- Irritability and staff conflict
- Insomnia
- Depression
- Substance and alcohol use
- Poor personal health
- Relationship difficulties
- Loss of work-life balance

Assessment—The Clinician and The Workplace

When assessing for burnout, focus needs to be directed at both the individual and the workplace setting.

Risk and Protective Factors

The range of responses outlined in the background section remind us of the importance of factors that can modify or mitigate the impact for clinicians (protective factors), while also understanding those factors that increase the likelihood of significant distress and adverse health outcomes among palliative care clinicians (risk factors). Consideration of both risk and protective factors can provide insights into opportunities for interventions that can support and promote the well-being of clinicians.[2]

At the individual level, clinicians will bring with them to their clinical work their personal life experience (including especially relevant experiences such as past losses and illness experience in self or others, and established coping responses), and their spiritual and cultural perspectives on dying. When the care for a dying patient resonates with past or current adversity in a clinician's life, and when personal emotional demands weigh heavily on the clinician, distress and difficulties coping can escalate.

The confrontation with death, suffering, and the limitations of curative treatments can challenge a clinician's professional identity and aspirations, and present a challenge to the clinician's own adaptation to death anxiety, sometimes referred to as "existential maturity," being able to appreciate one's own mortality without being overwhelmed by fear and loss.[6] These can become potent sources of distress and demoralization, contributing to a loss of personal meaning and purpose for the clinician. The emotional load met through confrontation with a patient's existential concerns can be compounded by an often cited sense of "not knowing what to say" to patients expressing such distress or concerns. Personal resilience or "hardiness" can be protective and reflected in the capacity to maintain a sense of commitment, purpose, and control in the face of these deeply challenging situations. Maintaining a robust network of social supports and strength of attachments outside of the clinical role can help create greater balance, and provide other sources of personal reward, self-esteem, and connection with others that is protective against the stress of this work.

Specific patient characteristics might heighten the risk of adverse impact on clinicians[7] and include:—

- Patients whose personal characteristics foster a clinician's closer personal identification with them (e.g., age, background or culture, type of illness, or patients who are health professionals);
- Where the patient had conflicted relationships with previous clinicians or perceived failures in care by clinical teams, thus creating greater mistrust by the patient or family;
- Patients whose reactions and responses are especially challenging in a way that undermines the rewards of engagement with the patient through their care.

The clinical and ethical challenges faced by clinicians in addressing treatment decisions and priorities in end of life care are further heightened by the growing focus in some regions on euthanasia and assisted suicide (see also Chapter 6), especially where this may cause conflict within clinical teams and for individual clinician's values. Professionals´ attitude toward death may also influence their well-being, as well as the quality of care they can offer to terminally ill patients and their families.

The challenges faced in caring for some specific clinical conditions may increase the risk among clinicians and teams, e.g., those conditions that are particularly distressing and place greater physical and emotional demands on clinicians over an extended period of disease or are confronting through disfigurement (either by the disease or the necessary treatment, such as in advanced head and neck cancer).

Children and younger patients, whose illness and its demands are even more untimely in the life cycle, or patients who have younger children themselves, can be especially challenging for clinicians. Patients or families with whom clinicians and teams have an especially close or long-standing relationship over the course of their illness can engender greater distress and grief;[7] while these may be realistic and human emotions to have, they become problematic if they impact on the clinicians' abilities to maintain usual care practices.

The Clinical Workplace

Consideration also needs to be given to the organizational environment of clinical care. Effective clinical leadership and governance is essential to promote the well-being of clinical staff as a core responsibility of health services, not only to meet obligations to those staff but as a key ingredient to the best possible patient care. These essential leadership responsibilities encompass policies and practices that address a commitment to staff well-being, encourage clinician participation in decision-making, ensure access to appropriate support when needed, and monitor workload and demands.

Professional skill development: Such leadership prioritizes continuing education to ensure skills match the demands of the clinical roles in palliative care:

• providing the opportunity for clinicians to remain up-to-date,
• to receive beneficial supervision of their work,
• to reflect on their practice, and
• to communicate a clear and consistent framework of values and agreed guidelines for practice.

A *workplace culture* that promotes respectful team-work is essential to supporting work satisfaction and the ability to navigate the sometimes complex clinical challenges in end of life care with a sense of purpose, collegiality, and personal reward. A valuable element of multidisciplinary care and team support can be the sharing of common values, supporting each other in the burden and emotional load of often difficult and complex tasks in care, and shared responsibility for individual patient care, scaffolded by effective leadership and accountability.

Protective factors can also include those strategies that

• promote effective boundaries between the work of palliative care and other aspects of the clinician's life;
• through realistic workload expectations, attention to rostering and vacation practices; and
• through leadership that communicates the importance of work-life balance.

Clinicians should be encouraged to maintain a wider repertoire of interests, where a robust sense of professional identity is balanced by a personal identity of a wider connected social network and other roles (such as family roles, leisure interests, and community contributions). Working in palliative care can provide a strong sense of identity, purpose, and wider societal value, often reinforced by a positive regard and social recognition for undertaking this work. Such recognition can also assist in sustaining the demands, but needs to be balanced by a realistic acknowledgment of these demands.

The support for clinicians to reflect on and identify this emotional impact, understand its effects on themselves and the care provided to the patient, and seek collegial advice and professional guidance can be helpful ingredients to promoting resilience. Such collegial guidance and formal mechanisms for review of more complex or challenging clinical or ethical dilemmas encountered in palliative care are likely to be beneficial.

In addition to supporting these healthy work practices, a workplace culture can be protective through promoting skill development: this includes being open to staff development needs, identifying gaps and nonjudgmental support for staff to acquire new skills when it is evident that these are needed. The most commonly cited needs in palliative care are skills in communication, including patient-family and internal team interactions. Guidelines exist that can help clinicians in responding to a number of the challenges in end of life communication, including discussing treatment goals, maintaining realistic hope, and discussing death.[8]

Other organizational risk factors include working in smaller, more isolated teams, working long hours, or working in isolation chiefly in home-care settings without the benefit of team-based support, guidance and collegiality.

Management Approaches

Despite the scope of the problems outlined above, evidence regarding efficacy of interventions is limited. Nevertheless, it is generally agreed that any interventions need to be multilevel in nature, giving attention to both individual and organizational factors, within a context of supportive leadership and workplace practices.[9]

Strategies that primarily address the needs of individuals, have focussed on building "resilience," an adaptability to many of the inevitable stressors in palliative care.[2] A "scaffolding" for individuals through a skills-based focus, with an emphasis on building self-reflection to respond to day-to-day work demands, includes emotional regulation (such as "mindfulness" practices), maintaining healthy boundaries, reasonable expectations, and other cognitive strategies.[2] These have the potential to prevent burnout in this setting.[10] Focus on attention regulation and the acceptance that characterize the use of these techiques have been shown to reduce distress, improve psychological well-being, foster resilience and spiritual well-being, and strengthen a prosocial motivation in patient encounters.[11]

Staff Support Programs

The concept of "staff support" can extend from informal discussions, which occur on a day-to-day basis, through to structured and formally facilitated staff support interventions.

- The routine use of formal "critical incident stress debriefing" in clinical settings is not well supported by evidence and may in some instances lead to negative outcomes.[12] Opportunities to promote sharing of clinical experience, reflection, and learning (e.g., Balint groups) can facilitate coping, support, and build clinical understanding and confidence.
- Sharing the grief that frequently arises in the palliative care setting may reduce the burden of caring for the dying and help staff work through the losses.
- Staff members may be offered noncompulsory, structured group meetings to memorialize patients that have died (see Box 11.1). Such meetings should respect the need to participate and disclose. More elaborate group

> **Box 11.1 Key Questions and Strategies to Support Staff**
>
> - What made things easy or difficult in his/her care?
> - What the staff member learned from caring for such a patient?
> - Sharing the experience of patient loss may also take place during established clinical sessions, i.e., multidisciplinary rounds, where a few minutes can be dedicated to mention specific aspects of the care of patients that have recently died.
> - Clinical discussions that employ a "grand rounds" case review from multiple perspectives and seek to identify issues of communication and compassionate care provision.

meetings may be led by a staff member briefly summarizing the medical history and circumstances of the patient´s death and facilitating the disclosure of those professionals who choose to share their experience and memories of the patient and family.

Any creative way of helping work through the grief that arises from continued exposure to loss and death will be helpful when offered as an option and when adjusted to staff members´ needs.

Stigma surrounding mental health problems is widespread among health professionals, and a frequent barrier to seeking professional guidance when needed. Support to seek professional assessment and treatment when concerns about depression, anxiety, substance use, or other clinical disorders exist, is essential. An organizational culture that promotes early intervention and ready access to such help, understanding the personal and professional barriers that might exist among clinicians to seeking such help, is a key element of a healthy clinical workplace. Chaplaincy services can provide an important source of support for many staff. Most importantly, workplace policies need to promote trust, respect professional boundaries, and protect clinicians' need for confidentiality. When psychiatric or psychological assessment and treatment is needed, this should not be provided within the staff members' own institution, where confidentiality is more difficult to guarantee. Timely external referral processes may be needed. Workplace policies are needed that assist and guide clinical managers to address these sometimes challenging situations, while supporting the clinicians, and maintaining the quality of patient care, which risks being impacted by unaddressed impairment in clinicians.

Education and Skill Development

Frameworks to guide clinical care at the end of life are a valuable source of assistance and support for clinicians. These frameworks can serve to guide them in engagement around existential concerns and can provide clinicians with the tools to communicate, understand, and respond to the patients concerns, exemplified by those strategies focusing on fostering patient's dignity and the exploration of personal meaning or spirituality for patients.[13,14]

Communication Issues

In palliative care, the evidence consistently points to the importance of skills in communication, negotiation around sometimes complex decisions for patients, families, and clinical teams, and skills in responding to the distress and suffering of patients and families.[12] When job demands exceed available resources, the risk to well-being is elevated. Such resources refer not only to adequate staffing levels, but importantly to factors such as support from superiors, appropriate decision authority, rewards, and coworker support.

Significant challenges can exist for clinicians working within smaller and more remote communities, such as rural areas, where the boundaries between professional and personal life are more difficult to maintain (e.g., where social and family connections within the community may exist), and where it can be difficult to exercise realistic boundaries in work demands, especially where a sense of community responsibility is paramount.

Professional Issues and Service Implementation

Ethical Issues

Moral distress: The concept of "moral injury" and "moral distress" has become a useful framework for considering the impact of an increasingly complex clinical environment in palliative care—with complex treatment or care decisions and varying cultural, legal, and professional frameworks that might surround the clinician, especially where these might feel in conflict with personal values. This tension has been intensified for many clinicians through the COVID-19 pandemic, as they confront risk of infection to oneself while undertaking their professional roles in patient care.

As public debate has grown in some countries regarding requests for assisted suicide, the emotional impact of such clinical and ethical dilemmas for practitioners caring for dying patients has also been a focus of attention (see also Chapter 6).

In the clinical context, responses to distressing events are thought to include four dimensions:

- accurate empathy (emotional attunement),
- perspective taking (cognitive attunement),
- memory (personal experience), and
- moral sensitivity (ethical attunement).

These dynamically intertwined dimensions create the preconditions for how clinicians respond to a triggering event instigated by an ethical conflict or dilemma. If the four dimensions are highly aligned, the intensity and valence of emotional arousal will influence ethical appraisal and discernment by engaging a robust view of the ethical issues, conflicts, and possible solutions and cultivating empathic action and resilience. In contrast, if they are not aligned, ethical appraisal and discernment will be deficient, creating emotional disregulation and potentially leading to personal and moral distress, self-focused behaviors, unregulated moral outrage, burnout, and secondary stress.[15] Moral distress develops when professionals cannot carry out what they believe to be ethically appropriate actions. It may negatively affect clinicians' well-being and job retention.

Clinical ethics committees can assist in guiding clinicians through some-times competing ethical demands and complex decisions (e.g., identifying and ceasing "futile" treatments; competing family and patient needs or requests). It is also important to recognise the sometimes unaddressed or unrecognized clinical issues (e.g., an unrecognized delirium or depression in a patient that contributes to team decision-making conflict) that can underpin what at first appears to be an ethical dilemma.

Teams and Supervision

Clinical supervision is well established in some disciplines and can provide a valuable source of professional guidance, validation and skill development in responding to such challenges.

Access to supervision (even if provided remotely) is important to ensure guidance in navigating these pressures, ideally with an understanding of the important local cultural and social factors. While such a role can be an important source of meaning and reward for the clinician in their community, it can also carry psychosocial risks to the clinician if demands become overly burdensome and managed in isolation from team-based support.

Culture and Service Delivery Issues

The following section aims to consider the issues for care providers in varying international contexts, with a specific focus on low resourced settings, as illus-trated through the development of the provision of community-based care and support for these carers.

Care in the Low Resource Cultural Context

The palliative and end of life care in Sub-Saharan Africa is an obstacle course.[16] It leads to a much larger perspective than the simple diagnosis of the disease, because it creates a moral obligation to care for human beings.[17] The care of the illness requires attention not only to the physical but also includes the so-ciocultural and spiritual environment of the patient and his/her family, which must be taken into account in the smallest details.

In the setting of Rwanda, after the genocide against the Tutsis in 1994, when one million people lost their lives and the sense of humanity was obso-lete, there was no longer a health system, let alone an appropriate model of palliative care for the country. A new approach was needed to build better quality of life for the population, especially at the end of life.

One approach developed by the government was to have the health serv-ices operate at the level of the community, but the challenges were huge.[18] The low number of doctors and nurses in the hospitals did not facilitate the task. It was necessary to draw on preexisting community practices, engaging people already integrated within the community with a certain level of ed-ucation, in a role recognized and designed by peers to be a bridge between communities and the community health workers.

One of the lessons learned during the course of this project was how to use existing practices and community resources to develop an adaptive and sustainable model of care. Introducing another system could be costly and inefficient for the quality of life and perception of care of patients and their families. This has been instructive in learning to listen more to the people to ensure sustainability, rather than to come up with an innovative model, developed in another context and adapted poorly.

The health workers were already very well recognized as effective people in their community, which was an important social recognition, but the logistics were also important. The advantage of this model was that it harnessed an existing model of care, using people who know the patients and whom they trust; the relationship between the health centers and the villages allowed for participation collectively, and it proved more likely to be adopted by the villages and hence be sustainable.

In Kigali, in 2010, 498 community health workers (CHWs) (one per village) were trained to support end of life care at the household level. There was no specific program for these nonmedical personnel at the time, so defining the role and care that they would provide within the home was difficult. Training was conducted over a day in groups of up to 20 people, addressing two main points: identification and assessment of pain (simple, moderate, and severe) and reporting on those people who require palliative care. These community health workers were to be the "eyes and ears" of the doctors. Their role focused on five conditions [Cancers, HIV/AIDS, heart disease, renal failure, and progressive neurological diseases] to better identify palliative care needs in their villages.

Two health center nurses from each village were also trained to support community health workers for rapid intervention. The nurses played a supervisory role and helped with the transfer of patients as needed. The person in charge of the community health workers also helped to report to the hospital's palliative care team using both a case identifier and pain level. This connection from the village to the hospital, which ensured patients, families, community health workers, and the hospital palliative care team supported each other, enabled case discussions, identifying any difficulties and opportunities to continue supporting patients in their local villages.

A case example illustrates this community-based model of care.

Case Study

Her name was Josiane M., a girl of 9 years, whom the community health workers had sent for palliative care support to one of the hospitals in Kigali, Rwanda, that was the first to be trained in palliative care. Josiane was suffering with a large tumor on her left eye. The Community Health Worker played a critical role in connecting Josiane to the hospital.

Josiane's mother described that Josiane had been the subject of mockery in the village and the school because of her disfigurement, and that Josiane had withdrawn, did not play with other children, nor go to the school. Tears of pain and suffering started to flow from the mother's eyes, but she maintained a serene face because she didn't want to show any sign of weakness. After the intervention of the palliative care team, Josiane was able to be sent to Kabgayi, where she received plastic surgery.

A few months after this surgical operation at Kabgayi hospital, Josiane and her mother came back to the local hospital to meet the staff. Josiane was happier, smiled, and played. For the nursing staff, seeing Josiane without this large tumor over her left eye and no longer needing to hide behind her mother, and hearing the impact of the treatment that made life possible again for Josiane, enabled the team to turn the sorrow into joy. This encouraged the community health workers to continue their work at the village level. Her mother declared: "In my opinion, [watching] Josiane smile again after several years, play with the other children, and go to school was the greatest gift that God has given me through you. God bless you."

Josiane's case inspired the palliative care team. They experienced a feeling of satisfaction because their training made it possible to identify patients through the community health workers. They had also carried a feeling of guilt because Josiane's case was discovered at an advanced stage. They realized that an earlier intervention would have been beneficial.

In the Rwandan social context, it is said, *"When you are well, you belong to yourself but when you are sick, you belong to your family."* This principle is understood within the model of patient decision-making and community involvement. Above all, it was important to learn, [and not just to teach] how community health workers deal with the psychological aspects present in the care of dying patients. The community is an important source of psychological support (sharing, discussions, parables, tales, proverbs, etc.). Given the cultural perception of death as a journey and not an end, it is possible to better manage losses in the community. It creates a sense of meaning and purpose in their work that helps cope with the demands of caring for dying patients. The philosophy behind this model of care is *"Ubuntu,"* which is rooted in African society and can be translated as *"I am because of you"* or *"people are people through other people."*[18] This African philosophy makes it possible to understand that it is all about the human being and our sense of humanity which stretches beyond the government's financing structures.

The end of life model differs from country to country, from culture to culture, and yet accessibility and availability of services are vital. It is crucial to take into account the cultural perception of life and death in the local context in order to develop a model of care that is equitable and respectful of local values and the values of the community workers—so the model reflects community values and accords with community workers' culture. Many models of care in Africa come from a Western culture that is costly to Africa, based on continuous funding and built on policies that are not related to the context. For example, the approach to autonomy, i.e., the patient in a developed country decides everything, is totally different in the context of Sub-Saharan Africa.

In the experience at the end of life in Rwanda, it was also important to know that the genocide survivors should have a model of care sensitive to the trauma they suffered and all the stress that was entailed. The Rwandan philosophy about the personal expression of feelings is Stoicism, which is a sociocultural value based on resilience and being able to endure suffering to find meaning in life. The idea that sadness must be half-expressed, half-hidden is omnipresent in Rwandan culture. One Rwandan expression describes this reality very well: "*Amalira y'umugabo atemba ajya mu nda*" (In Rwanda, tears flow within).

It was critical to draw guidance initially from other approaches and be inspired with the experience of several international experts who have worked within developing countries, such as Partners in Health (PIH), working with local governments and communities to improve health through biopsychosocial perspectives.[19] In the end of life context, support is needed outside the hospital setting, requiring a broad model of care involving family, community, and volunteers, drawing inspiration from their existing practices. A good example is task-shifting: giving greater responsibility to nurses, helping reduce reliance on hospitals, and the resulting physical and financial burden for patients and families.

It was necessary to have a local care *system* and model adapted to the sociocultural context—a model that identifies the needs of patients and their families at the end of life, focusing on the patient and the community with approaches relevant to the local context rather than adopting conventional global models. Standardization of models can perpetuate social injustice if it disregards the local perceptions and needs.

In Africa, the community remains and will always remain the best *space* for the support of the patient and his family at the end of life, with the understanding of the sociocultural aspects of the patient's ecosystem. The alignment between the local knowledge and resources, and with a culture shared by Community Health Workers, helps support those in these roles.

Rwanda and other African countries have understood the importance of investing in human capital to improve the service and the quality of care for vulnerable populations at the end of life. Africa has shared a lot in terms of the experience regarding the role of community-based human resources and community involvement. Developed countries could also learn from the good practices of developing countries through this global perspective.

Conclusion

Providing care at the end of life presents a range of professional and personal challenges for clinicians. These are often balanced against the personal rewards of providing care to the dying patient and their family. Symptoms such as depression, anxiety, demoralization and what is sometimes referred to as "burnout" can occur among clinicians when demands overwhelm the rewards. Factors that can contribute to the emotional load of such work include cumulative grief, coping with the limitations of curative treatments, refocusing goals, and the often clinical and ethical complexity of care. Other relevant factors can include the risk and protective factors at the personal level of the clinician, through to the factors in the organization and culture of the clinical workplace itself.

Interventions to support clinicians include those that ensure clinicians are appropriately prepared with the necessary skills and supported in their roles, effective mentorship and supervision, strong leadership and teamwork that promotes support and clinician well-being, and steps to promote a sense of meaning and purpose in this work.

Cultural factors, and the varying models of care relevant to different settings globally need to be considered, including the critical role of community workers in provision of appropriate and effective end of life care in diverse locations.

References

1. Melvin CS. Historical review in understanding burnout, professional compassion fatigue, and secondary traumatic stress disorder from a hospice and palliative nursing perspective. J Hosp Palliat Nurs. 2015;17(1):66–72.

2. Back AL, Steinhauser KE, Kamal AH, Jackson VA. Building resilience for palliative care: An approach to burnout prevention based on individual skills and workplace factors. J Pain Sympt Manage. 2016;52:284–291.

3. Dijxhoom AF, Brom L, van der Linden Y, et al. Prevalence of burnout in healthcare professionals providing palliative care and the effect of interventions to reduce symptoms: A systematic literature review. Palliat Med. 2021;35(1):6–26.

4. Renzenbrink I. Staff support: Whose responsibility? Grief Matters. 2005;8:13–17.

5. Venes D, ed. Taber's cyclopedic medical dictionary. 23rd ed. Philadelphia, PA: F.A. Davis Pub; 2013. Pages 526, 902, 1147–1148, 1740.

6. Emmanuel L, Solomon S, Fitchett G, et al. Fostering existential maturity to manage terror in a pandemic. J Palliat Med. 2021;24(2):211–217.

7. Meier DE, Back AL, Morrison RS. The inner life of physicians and care of the seriously ill. JAMA. 2001;286:3007–3014.

8. Clayton JM, Hancock K, Butow PN et al. Clinical practice guidelines for communicating prognosis and end of life issues with adults in the advanced stages of a life-limiting illness, and their caregivers. Med J Aust. 2007;186(12): S77–S108.

9. Harrison KL, Dzeng E, Ritchie C, et al. Addressing palliative care clinician burnout in organizations: A workforce necessity, an ethical imperative. J Pain Sympt Manage. 2017;53(6):1091–1096.

10. Fillion L, Vachon M, Gagnon P. Enhancing meaning at work and preventing burnout: The meaning-centered intervention for palliative care clinicians. In Breitbart W, Editor. Meaning-Centered Psychotherapy in the Cancer Setting: Finding Meaning and Hope in the Face of Suffering. New York: Oxford University Press; 2017. Pages 168–181.

11. Orellana-Rios CL, Radbruch L, Kern M, et al. Mindfulness and compassion-oriented practices at work reduce distress and enhance self-care of palliative care teams: A mixed-method evaluation of an "on the job" program. BMC Palliative Care 2018;17:3.

12. Turner J, Kelly B, Girgis A. Supporting Oncology Health Professionals: A Review. Psychooncologie. 2011;5:77–82.

13. Breitbart W, Pessin H, Rosenfeld B, et al. Individual meaning-centred psychotherapy for the treatment of psychological and existential distress: A randomized controlled trial in patients with advanced cancer. Cancer. 2018;124(15):3231–3239.

14. Sinclair S, Chochinov HM. Communicating with patients about existential and spiritual issues: SACR-D work. Prog Palliat Care. 2012;20(2):72–78.

15. Rushton C, Kaszniak A, Halifax J. A framework for understanding moral distress among palliative care clinicians. J Pall Med. 2013;16(9):1074–1079.

16. Harding R, Higginson IJ. Palliative care in sub-Saharan Africa. Lancet. 2005;365(9475):1971–1977. https://doi.org/10.1016/S0140-6736(05)66666-4.

17. Krakauer EL, Rajagopal MR. End of life care across the world: A global moral failing. Lancet. 2013;388(10043):444–446. https://doi.org/10.1016/S0140-6736(16)31133-3.

18. Ntizimira CR, Ngizwenayo S, Krakauer EL, Dunne ML, Esmaili E. Addressing end of life care in cancer patients through "Ubuntu": Lessons learned from Rwanda in global health perspective of humanity. Curr Obst Gynec Reports. 2016;5(4):273–278. https://doi.org/10.1007/s13669-016-0186-7.

19. Aziz, R. Battling TB and other outbreaks: "staff, stuff, space, and systems" still lacking. Science Speaks: Global ID News. 2016, March 22. https://sciencespeaksblog.org/2016/03/22/tb-survivor-i-assumed-id-be-okay/.

Further Reading

Meier DE, Back AL, Morrison RS. The inner life of physicians and care of the seriously ill. JAMA. 2001;286:3007–3014. This review provides a comprehensive and practical summary of the personal and clinical factors that can contribute to the challenges clinicians face in the care of seriously ill patients, with useful indicators of those clinical situations that can present greater risk to clinicians and practical recommendations to support clinicians.

Back AL, Steinhauser KE, Kamal AH, Jackson VA. Building resilience for palliative care: An approach to burnout prevention based on individual skills and workplace factors. J Pain Sympt Manage. 2016;52:284–291. This article will provide readers with a framework for considering the common features of burnout, factors contributing to stress among palliative care clinicians, and practical strategies to both prevent and address burnout in this setting.

Clayton JM, Hancock K, Butow PN, et al. Clinical practice guidelines for communicating prognosis and end of life issues with adults in the advanced stages of a life-limiting illness, and their caregivers. Med J Aust. 2007;186(12):S77–S108. Communication with patients and families about key issues in is a common source of stress for palliative care clinicians. This publication will provide readers with evidence based guidance on addressing these challenges in communication at the end of life.

Example of a Question Prompt List for Palliative Care[1]

The following are common questions that people with life-threatening illnesses sometimes ask their doctors. Please indicate the ones that you may like to ask today and the doctors will do their best to answer them.

About the Palliative Care Team and Service

1. What does the palliative care service offer that is different from services provided by the other doctors/nurses that I see?
2. What is the role of my GP now that I have been referred to the palliative care team?

Physical Symptoms

1. If I have symptoms, what can be done to improve them? (e.g., pain or discomfort, constipation, shortness of breath, nausea or feeling sick, lack of appetite, tiredness, dry mouth)
2. What is the cause of my symptoms?

Treatment

1. Are there any medications that I should stop taking because of their interactions with the newly prescribed medication?
2. Are there any natural or complementary (alternative) therapies that may be helpful for me?

Lifestyle and Quality of Life

1. Can you advise me about the timing of a holiday or trip I wish to take?
2. How can I remain close and intimate with my partner (physically and/or emotionally)?

My Illness and What to Expect in the Future

1. What are the chances of controlling my illness? Will the illness progress?
2. How long am I likely to live?

Support

1. Is there someone I can talk to about my fears and concerns?
2. What support is available for other people in the family, e.g., carer or my children?

End of life Issues

1. Who can I talk to about the medical care that I want in the future when I am no longer able to speak for myself?
2. Is it feasible for me to die at home rather than in the palliative care ward or hospital?

For Carers

1. Can I get help if I cannot manage?
2. What should I say when the person that I am caring for asks, "Am I dying"?

Reference

1. Abridged with permission from Asking Questions Can Help: An Aid for People Seeing the Palliative Care Team (Clayton J, Butow P, Tattersall M, et al. Asking questions can help: Development and preliminary evaluation of a question prompt list for palliative care patients. Br J Cancer. 2003;89(11):2069–2077. https://doi.org/10.1038/sj.bjc.6601380).

Appendix 2

Example of an Advance Care Plan

Your Personal Details	
Unique Patient Identifier:	
Surname:	
Given name:	
Date of Birth:	

Part 1: Appointment of a Medical Treatment Decision Maker and Support Person

Your medical treatment decision maker has legal authority to make medical decisions on your behalf, if you do not have decision-making capacity to make the decision. The second person you list will only be asked if the first person is unavailable.

I appoint as my medical treatment decision maker(s):

Medical Treatment Decision Maker 1	
Full Name:	
Date of Birth:	
Address:	
Phone Number:	
Acceptance of Appointment: I understand the obligations of an appointed Medical Treatment Decision Maker and undertake to act in accordance with any known preferences and values of the person making the appointment. I undertake to promote the personal and social well-being of the person making the appointment and have read and understand any advance care directive that the person has given.	
Name: Signature: Date:	

Medical Treatment Decision Maker 2	
Full Name:	
Date of Birth:	
Address:	
Phone Number:	
Acceptance of Appointment: I understand the obligations of an appointed Medical Treatment Decision Maker and undertake to act in accordance with any known preferences and values of the person making the appointment. I undertake to promote the personal and social well-being of the person making the appointment and have read and understand any advance care directive that the person has given.	
Name: Signature: Date:	

Witness to Appointment of Medical Treatment Decision Maker(s)	
Witness 1	Witness 2
Name:	Name:
Signature:	Signature:
Date:	Date:

Part 2: Values Directive

We are all unique and have different beliefs, values, and goals. Here you can say what is important to you. What does it mean to you to "live well"? This information will be used by people making decisions for you to help them make the decisions that you would have made yourself. These statements are a guide to treatment decision-making only. If you wish to legally refuse treatment, see Part 3 of this form.

You may complete all, some or none of the sections:

What matters most in my life: (what does living well mean to you)	
What worries me most about my future:	
For me unacceptable outcomes of medical treatment after illness or injury are: (e.g., loss of independence, high-level care, or not being able to recognize people or communicate)	
Other things I would like known are:	
Other people I would like involved in decisions about my care:	
If I am nearing death the following things would be important to me: (e.g., where I would prefer to die, spiritual/faith rituals or requests, who I would like with me, funeral preferences)	

Part 3: Instructional Directive

This instructional directive is legally binding and communicates your medical treatment decision(s) directly to your health practitioner(s). It is recommended that you consult a medical practitioner if you choose to complete this instructional directive.

- Your instructional directive will only be used if you do not have decision-making capacity to make a medical treatment decision.
- Your medical treatment decisions in this instructional directive take effect as if you had consented to, or refused to, begin or continue medical treatment.
- If your Instructional Directives are unclear, they will still be considered as descriptions of your values.

I CONSENT to the following treatment: (specify medical treatment and the circumstances)	
I REFUSE the following treatment: (specific medical treatment and the circumstances)	
Cardiopulmonary Resuscitation (CPR) involves chest compressions and artificial ventilation to manually save brain function, blood circulation, and breathing for someone in cardiac arrest. These interventions are used when a person's heart stops beating, and they may or may not restore life.	If my heart stops beating: ☐ Attempt resuscitation if clinically indicated ☐ Do NOT attempt resuscitation Comment:
Organ donation: Very few people die in a way that allows them to be considered for organ donation. One organ donor can save or improve the lives of many others. Your family will be asked to confirm your consent for donation.	In the event that I am able to be considered for organ, eye and/or tissue donation when I die, I wish to be a donor: ☐ Yes ☐ No Comment:

Part 4: Witnessing and Signature

Your declaration: I make this Advance Care Directive and any appointments within it freely and voluntarily, and I understand the nature and effect of each statement within the Plan.

Name:	
Signature:	
Date:	

Witnesses to the signing of this Advance Care Plan: I certify that the person giving this Advance Care Plan appears to have decision-making capacity and has freely and voluntarily signed the document in the presence of two witnesses, neither of whom has been appointed as a Medical Treatment Decision Maker. The person appears to understand the nature and effect of all statements made within this document.

Witness 1: Registered Medical Practitioner	Witness 2
Name:	Name:
Signature:	Signature:
Date:	Date:
Qualifications:	

Appendix 3

Demoralization Scale-II (DS-II)[1]

For each statement below, please indicate how much (or how strongly) you have felt this way **over the last two weeks** by circling the corresponding number. **Here are some statements about your morale.**

	Never	Some-times	Often
1. There is little value in what I can offer others.	0	1	2
2. My life seems to be pointless.	0	1	2
3. My role in life has been lost.	0	1	2
4. I no longer feel emotionally in control.	0	1	2
5. No one can help me.	0	1	2
6. I feel that I cannot help myself.	0	1	2
7. I feel hopeless.	0	1	2
8. I feel irritable.	0	1	2
9. I do not cope well with life.	0	1	2
10. I have a lot of regret about my life.	0	1	2
11. I feel distressed about what is happening to me.	0	1	2
12. I am not a worthwhile person.	0	1	2
13. I would rather not be alive.	0	1	2
14. I feel quite isolated and alone.	0	1	2
15. I tend to feel hurt easily.	0	1	2
16. I feel trapped by what is happening to me.	0	1	2

Reference

1. Reproduced with permission from Robinson S, Kissane DW, Brooker J, et al. Refinement and revalidation of the Demoralization Scale: The DS-II—Internal validity. Cancer 2016;122:2251–2259. https://doi.org/10.1002/cncr.30015.

Appendix 4

Psycho-Existential Symptom Assessment Scale (PeSAS)[1]

Choose a number between 0 to 10 that tells us how bothered, worried or distressed you are by each symptom listed here.

Clinician to write the score under each date of assessment.

Record Date						
Anxiety						
Discouragement						
Trapped by illness						
Hopelessness						
Pointlessness						
Loss of control						
Loss of roles						
Depression						
Wish to die						
Confusion						

Reference

1. Adapted with permission from Kissane DW. Education and assessment of psycho-existential symptoms to prevent suicidality in cancer care. Psycho-Oncology. 2020;29(9). https://doi.org/10.1002/pon.5519.

Index

Tables, figures, and boxes are indicated by t, f, and b following the page number